LINKING MEDICAL CARE AND COMMUNITY SERVICES

Practical Models for Bridging the Gap

Walter Leutz, Ph.D., is an Associate Professor at Brandeis University's Heller School, where he teaches courses in long-term care. He is the Director of the Social HMO Consortium, a university-provider cooperative that has developed, expanded, and researched a managed care model for integrating acute and long-term care services for Medicare beneficiaries. He is also Research Director of a system-wide Kaiser Permanente demonstration of how to add community long-term care services to the Kaiser Permanente clinical continuum. Recent articles include "Caregiver education and support: Results of a multi-site pilot in an HMO" Home Health Services Quarterly, 2002, "A community care entitlement in the Social HMO: How members use services." *Journal of Aging and Social Policy,* 2001, and "Five laws for integrating medical and social care: Lessons from the US and UK," *Milbank Quarterly,* 1999. Dr. Leutz is also primary author of two other books on the practical development of coordinated community health care systems for elders: *Changing Health Care for An Aging Society* (1985), *Care for Frail Elders* (1992).

Merwyn R. Greenlick, Ph.D., is professor emeritus and past chair of the Department of Public Health and Preventive Medicine, School of Medicine, Oregon Health & Sciences University. He also directs the Oregon Health Policy Institute. Until July, 1995, he was director of the Kaiser Permanente Center for Health Research (CHR) and Vice President for Research, Kaiser Foundation Hospitals. He was instrumental in starting the CHR in 1964 and was its director for more than 30 years. He has served as research advisor to many projects throughout the country and as an advisor to several foreign government research and medical care projects. He was elected to the Institute of Medicine of the National Academy of Sciences in 1971. Dr. Greenlick's research has been in the areas of large-scale demonstration projects relating to the organization and financing of medical care and behavioral interventions in disease prevention. He has also had extensive experience in clinical trials, both at the local and national levels, and has provided considerable leadership at the national level. Dr. Greenlick is a Distinguished Fellow of the Association for Health Services Research (now the Academy for Health Services Research and Health Policy) and, in 1994, received the Association's President's Award for his lifetime contributions to the field.

Lucy Nonnenkamp, MA, is currently the project director for the Kaiser Permanente Northwest's (KPNW) Social HMO, co-chairs KPNW's Senior and Disabled Care committee, and participates in the KPNW's Medicare visioning, strategic planning, oversight and operations functions. She coordinated the 1996 Kaiser Permanente Interregional Geriatric Institute and is currently on the Kaiser Permanente Aging Network Advisory committee. Ms. Nonnenkamp joined the Social HMO team in 1983 to write the in-home support benefit and case management component of the demonstration. She developed and supervised the expanded care department, which has oversight for the home and community-based long-term care benefit, until 1990. Ms. Nonnenkamp was the project administrator prior to becoming project director for the KPNW's Social HMO, locally marketed as Senior Advantage II.

Linking Medical Care and Community Services

Practical Models for Bridging the Gap

Walter Leutz, PhD
Merwyn R. Greenlick, PhD
Lucy Nonnenkamp, MA

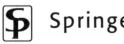 Springer Publishing Company

Springer Publishing Company, Inc.
536 Broadway
New York, NY 10012-3955

Acquisitions Editor: Sheri W. Sussman
Production Editor: Janice G. Stangel
Cover design by Joanne Honigman

03 04 05 06 07 / 5 4 3 2 1

Library of Congress Cataloging-in-Publication Data

Leutz, Walter N.
   Linking medical care and community services : practical models for
bridging the gap / Walter Leutz, Merwyn R. Greenlick, Lucy Nonnenkamp,
authors.
      p. cm.
   Includes bibliographic references and index.
   ISBN 0-8261-1754-6
   1. Long-term care of the sick. 2. Community health services. 3. Medical
care. I. Greenlick, Merwyn R. II. Nonnenkamp, Lucy. III. Title.

RA997 .L48 2003
362.1—dc21

2002030680

Printed in the United States of America by Sheridan Books.

Contents

Contributors

Alissa Au
Kaiser Permanente Honolulu Clinic
Honolulu, HI

Janet Bath
Program Consultant
Del Mar, CA

Pauline Bourgeois
Kaiser Permanente Mid-Atlantic
Rockville, MD

Kathy Brody
Kaiser Permanente Center
   for Health Research
Portland, OR

Aurora deJesus
Kaiser Permanente Ohio
Cleveland, OH

Richard DellaPenna
Kaiser Permanente Southern
   California
San Diego, CA

Marna Flaherty-Robb
Oregon Health Sciences University
Portland, OR

Carla Green
Kaiser Permanente Center
   for Health Research
Portland, OR

Michelle Hillier
Group Health Cooperative
Takoma, WA

Mark Hornbrook
Kaiser Permanente Center
   for Health Research
Portland, OR

Enid Hunkeler
Kaiser Permanente Division
   of Research
Oakland, CA

Linda Johns
Kaiser Permanente Northwest
Portland, OR

Connie Keyes
Kaiser Permanente Northwest
Portland, OR

Marlene McKenzie
Kaiser Permanente Senior Programs
Denver, CO

Hanh Nguyen
Kaiser Permanente Golden Gate
   Services Area
San Francisco, CA

Phillip Percy
Kaiser Permanente Social Services
Riverside, CA

Ed Thomas
Kaiser Permanente Program Office
Garfield Memorial Fund
Oakland, CA

Ingrid Venohr
Kaiser Permanente Geriatric
  Programs
Denver, CO

Nancy Vuckovic
Kaiser Permanente Center
  for Health Research
Portland, OR

Warren Wong
Kaiser Permanente Moanalua
  Medicine Center
Honolulu, HI

Preface

My interest in Medicare beneficiaries began in the summer of 1986, a few months after I assumed responsibility for the operation of Kaiser Permanente's Northwest Region. At the time, the Northwest Region was the only KP region to have an over-65 population which was representative of the elderly population in the community. Because the other KP regions were considering expanding their Medicare populations, the Northwest's experience was of great interest to them.

As a result, the Kaiser Permanente Committee, the policy-making body for the organization, established, and asked me to chair, an interdivisional group of managers, physicians, researchers, and advisors called the Medicare Task Force. This group was charged with addressing all of the issues related to Kaiser Permanente's long-term relationship with its elderly population and with Medicare. Among other things, the Medicare Task Force affirmed that all KP regions would achieve a share of Medicare beneficiaries proportionate to the communities they served. It also pointed out the need for ongoing committees to address the complex and evolving issues related to the care, and the financing of care, for these members.

This led to the formation of the Interregional Committee on Aging, the Medicare Policy and Finance Committee, and the Model of Care Committee. It was clear to everyone on these various committees, including several persons who contributed to this book, that the range and types of services provided to Medicare beneficiaries, how they were delivered, and how they were financed, were critically linked. To positively affect cost, outcomes, and quality-of-life issues, we needed to move to new models of care, some of which are outlined in this book.

Nearly 10 years later, my interest in caring for Medicare beneficiaries was rekindled from a very different perspective. My father, 85, living 3,000 miles away in Florida, legally blind and generally frail, fell and broke his hip. Happily, the immediate medical treatment of his problem was without incident. However, his prolonged stay in the skilled nursing facility following his discharge from the hospital began my immersion, and that of both of my parents, into the confusion and frustration of dealing with "the system." The complex rules governing what is covered and what is not (a function of

HMO coverage, physician orders, time between hospital discharge and admission to a SNF or hospital, what constitutes physical therapy, what constitutes a spell of illness, as well as other variables) were almost unfathomable, my experience as a health care executive notwithstanding.

During my many trips to Florida to help during his prolonged recovery period, another set of problems became apparent. My mother, 85 and in robust health, was becoming unable to carry out not only her expanded responsibilities as a care giver, but also activities that had been routine for her only months before. Getting to the doctors, keeping track of all of the medications (and learning the generics), knowing which medical statements needed to be paid and which didn't, as well as carrying out basic functions such as paying bills, shopping for food, cooking, and cleaning, were all becoming problematic.

Because they so treasured their independence, my parents continued to struggle with caring for themselves, with virtually no help from the community, for nearly four years. They finally accepted the often repeated offer of help from their children, and last summer moved from Florida to an assisted living facility in Oregon where extensive help was available and family was nearby. Still, some nagging questions remain: Were there resources in the community that we were unaware of that could have helped my parents? Would the decisions have been easier if my parents' health care system had known what was available in the community and had provided options not just for the medical care, but also for the support care they needed? Did the medical care system have the ability to connect me or my parents to community resources that could have lessened my parents struggle or improved their quality of life?

Although I am fortunate to have both 90-year-old parents alive and financially independent, and to have the time to devote to them, a knowledge of health care systems, and friends and colleagues in the medical community on whom I can call for help, I still find that navigating "the system" is sometimes a challenge. I can only imagine how difficult it is for the vast majority of American families who do not have these resources.

I hope that this book, which illustrates some ways to make "the system" easier to navigate, will help such families. The proposed models will not eliminate the challenges of being a caregiver or of having a disability, but they will establish clearer and more reliable ways for people to get help and information. Even though KP has done much since 1986 to improve its care systems for both the elderly and members with disabilities and chronic illnesses, the Manifesto 2005 demonstration shows that much remains to be done. More importantly, it shows that valuable changes are both feasible and affordable. Hopefully, KP and other health plans will find ways to adopt them.

MICHAEL H. KATCHER, PhD
President, Kaiser Foundation Health Plan of the Northwest (1986–1996)

Acknowledgments

This book was the work of many hands and minds and hearts, and we have tried to acknowledge as many as we can by showing our dependence on our coauthors for the project reports they wrote, the data they collected, and their careful reading, editing, and critique of our analyses and conclusions. In each chapter, we also acknowledge the larger project teams that worked for many months to conceive, plan, and implement the service and research projects that served so many members and their families.

Two unacknowledged individuals from the Center for Health Research in Portland, Oregon, deserve special credit: Catherine Janssen and Gary Miranda. Catherine was our expert, energetic, and upbeat assistant in arranging meetings, keeping track of reports, and logistics in general. Gary was once again a wise and supportive critic of our thinking and stylish editor of our first manuscript.

We also had the good fortune to work with Richard DellaPenna throughout the development, implementation, and evaluation of the demonstration. Richard's long experience as a geriatrician and medical leader within the Permanente Medical Group helped us improve the manuscript's clinical relevance.

Finally, the book was made possible when Ed Thomas, Director of the Garfield Memorial Fund, extended the evaluation contract to produce a more complete and coherent report on the demonstration. This allowed the many, many people who worked on this project within Kasier Permanente and in community care agencies to deepen their sense of accomplishment. We hope that this book soon leads to the reassembly of many of the old teams for another round of work on the important issues we identified, which are obviously far from resolved.

While the work rests on the shoulders of many, we take final responsibility for the interpretations, recommendations, and conclusions herein.

WALTER LEUTZ
MERWYN GREENLICK
LUCY NONNENKAMP

xi

Project Team Acknowledgments by Chapter

2 Manifesto 2005

Interregional Committee on Aging Chair: Toby Cole, MD.
Long-Term Care Committee: Richard DellaPenna, Glenn Gade,
    David Glass, Merwyn Greenlick (chair), Chris Himes,
    Lucy Nonnenkamp, Rik Smith, Neil Solomon, Elaine Welch,
    Warren Wong
Consultants: Marna Flaherty-Robb, Walter Leutz, Carl Serrato,
    Ed Thomas
Evaluation Team: Joyce Gilbert, Nancy Gordon, Merwyn Greenlick,
    Walter Leutz, Clyde Pope, Carl Serrato
Data Team: Kathy Brody, Jane Wallace

3 Reaching Out and Linking Up

Day Care: Edith Eddleman, Roy Jaffee, Michelle Hillier, Chris Himes,
    Eileen Lynette, Karen Lewis Smith, Ralph Yep
SF-CCP: Hanh Nguyen, Donna Schempp, Jeffery Sterman
Volunteers: David Cherry, Steve Graham, Jennifer Groebe,
    Anita Henning, Enid Hunkeler, Janell Lee, Marlene McKenzie,
    Adrienne Mims, Alexandria Shinn, Brenda Stevenson-Marshall,
    Barbara Warner, Ann Williams, Ralph Yep

4 Individuals with Disabilities and Their Families:
    Who Are They and What Helps Them Connect with Services?

Caregivers: Rida Ching, Marna Flaherty-Robb, Ilene Kasper,
    Wilhelmena Lee, Marlene McKenzie, Phillip Percy
Foster care: Kathy Brody, Arnold Hurtado, Connie Keyes,
    Linda VanBuren
NORCs: Alissa Au

5 Looking Inward: Making Change in Complex Organizations

Community health workers: Toni Africh, Janet Bath, Cherolyn Robertson
Temporary decline: Warren Wong
Adaptive equipment: Bunny Meharry, Linda Johns, Susan Kolibaba,
    Peg Macko, Debra Taylor
Dementia: Pauline Bourgeois, Debra Cherry, Douglas Connor,
    Richard DellaPenna, Robin Fine, Elizabeth Heck, Lynn Hodge,
    Maroni Leash, Marlene McKenzie, Lucy Nonnenkamp, Clyde Pope,
    Valisa Saunders, Catherine Steinbach, Elex Tenney, Vicki Vahan,
    Ingrid Venohr, Marilyn Williams

6 Infants, Children, and Non-elderly Adults with Disabilities

Disability event modeling: Kathleen Brody, Richard DellaPenna, Mark Hornbrook, Arnold Hurtado, John Pearson, John Stull
Younger disabled: Carla Green, Nancy Vucovic, Alison Firemark
Parents of children with disabilities: Marlene McKenzie, Elizabeth Romer, Ingrid Venohr
Vermont: Pauline Bourgeois, Ron Clark
Harvey: Aurora deJesus

Introduction

In the second half of the 20th Century the American medical care system emerged as a system for mitigating the consequences of acute care illnesses. The development of dramatic new diagnostic and treatment technologies accelerated the system's move away from focusing on "caring" for permanent disease toward a focus on "curing" episodes of illness. However, the graying of America and the increasing awareness of the impact of chronic disease and disability on American patients, especially the elderly, has begun to arrest this movement.

Nowhere has the situation become more apparent than in the organization and delivery of care within integrated care system HMOs such as Kaiser Permanente. These integrated care networks have the primary responsibility for the delivery of medical care (and perhaps even health care) services to an enrolled population. Consequently, they must explore balancing properly their investment in care and in cure. The investment consideration includes questions of health benefit components and questions of organizing and delivering clinical services.

Further, this question of balancing care and cure is especially complex when dealing with the portion of the population with known disabilities or with the most seriously disabling chronic illnesses. Because of the functional deficits of this population, it is not possible to meet their needs without the services generally available only outside of the boundaries of the typical medical care system. Therefore this dilemma is "writ large" when an integrated delivery system HMO begins to consider how to help disabled and chronically ill patients establish successful links with the providers of home- and community-based long-term care services.

Most medical care systems, even the very comprehensive ones, do not consider home- and community-based long-term care services (community care) within their clinical or coverage scope. Most physicians, even the most enlightened ones, do not feel that their professional responsibility extends to the day-in, day-out challenges of escalating disease and impairments, which lead to the need for community care. Yet, more and more, dedicated HMO clinical managers, physician and nursing leaders, are troubled by their inability to properly plan for and deliver services to this sub-set of the population.

This book addresses these issues, using experience and experiments from the largest of the integrated care system HMOs, Kaiser Permanente, to illuminate the discussion. Kaiser Permanente has been seriously addressing these questions for many years, through its national committee structure, its extensive aging services network, and its extraordinary historical predisposition to undertake public domain health services research to create knowledge.

The book asks the question "How can a medical care system structure itself to best serve the total care needs of the frail and disabled members of its population?" Addressing this question requires several steps. First we examine the nature of the two systems (medical care and long-term care) that these members must continually deal with. We explore alternative models of system integration. We report on an extraordinary 32-site demonstration program investigating the issues of linking the two systems for KP members. And finally, we synthesize these considerations to propose ways to facilitate the linking of these two systems in the future.

We believe the book will intrigue and challenge health care managers, geriatric and disability-oriented clinicians, health care educators, and the policy community. We have certainly enjoyed the privilege of digesting and presenting the work of a talented group of clinicians and researchers as a single, rich story and simple but powerful conceptual framework. The KP demonstration developed a provocative and innovative way to look at a problem that is proving to be increasingly vexing to the health care community, policy makers, and families around the nation.

WALTER LEUTZ
MITCH GREENLICK
LUCY NONNENKAMP

1

Coping with Aging and Disability

Walter Leutz

The experience that Michael Katcher relates in the Preface is ironic but by no means unusual: Even a medical professional can be stymied by the new experience of being a caregiver for an aging and disabled parent, spouse, or child. It is the rare person who has not had first-hand experience with helping a close friend or family member cope with chronic illness and disability. Most likely it's an aging parent or grandparent, but it may also be a working-age partner who has Multiple Sclerosis (MS), or who has been in an auto accident, or a baby born with Down Syndrome or cerebral palsy. The personal impacts of disability may be a mix of stress, loss, anger, physical and emotional pain, insight, financial strain, understanding, growth, reaffirmation, and more—both for disabled persons and their loved ones. Whether disability and chronic illness enter one's life suddenly or gradually, they also bring entry into new worlds of personally giving and receiving help, as well as finding and using help from a new universe of "helping" professions and organizations.

This book is about improving how "helping" professionals and organizations assist people in their struggles to cope with chronic illness and disability. It's about figuring out how to make disparate systems work together to make it easier for people to find services and use services effectively—on the one side medical care services such as doctors and hospitals, and on the other community care services such as personal care, homemakers, day center services, group homes, and transportation. Help from both of these sectors—medical care and community care—are usually essential to persons with disabilities, but they often operate as if they were in parallel universes.

The lack of communication and cooperation across medical and community care borders not only reduces the effectiveness of each but also complicates the already complicated lives of the vulnerable people they serve.

Most help for most people with disabilities is provided by families free of charge out of love and obligation, and much is also done by friends who do many small things, not the least of which is to just continue being a friend in spite of changes in functioning. More and more help is provided at home, and this is the way most people prefer it. Only the most disabled with the weakest family supports end up in institutions these days. Society has come a long way in changing its understanding and acceptance of disability and trying to provide the supports people with disabilities want to be independent and integrated in society. But there is still a long way to go.

A big part of the problem is facing up to the magnitude of the need and the nature of the problems and to the fact that the needs are sure to grow dramatically in coming decades. On the community care side, perhaps the biggest problem is that there is just too little funding—most spending is eaten up by institutional services. And what community care funds there are too often go to services that are not coordinated with one another. Services are typically under-funded, fragmented, means-tested, and uncoordinated. It's up to people with disabilities and their families to figure out what's available, if it's what they need, and how to pay for it.

On the medical side, for those with insurance (and most people with disabilities can get insurance through either Medicare or Medicaid) there is plenty of funding for increasingly complex and costly procedures, but projections of those costs are downright scary. At the same time, surprisingly little is done to accommodate the special needs of people with disabilities, (e.g., higher pay for longer office visits, special help with transportation, payment for geriatric services).

This book explores some new ways for the medical care system and the community care system to work together more closely and effectively to help people with chronic illnesses and disabilities. It eschews the currently popular notion of "integrating" medical and community care. Integration is a compelling concept since its goal is to overcome the problems of fragmentation and under funding of community care by pooling funds and putting a single agency in charge of a broad system of benefits and services. The idea to be proposed is that integration is a good idea in some circumstances and for some people, but for most people a simpler model that more closely links existing agencies across the borders of medical and community care systems is preferable.

On one level, this book is the story of why and how Kaiser Permanente (KP), America's oldest and largest group practice-model Health Maintenance Organization (HMO), tested ways to expand its mission to include community care services for its members with disabilities. Managed care organizations such as KP have traditionally created integrated delivery models for the treatment of acute illnesses for their members. As their members have aged, and as disability and chronic illness among other populations have increased in importance, the best HMOs have begun to develop chronic illness management protocols and extended geriatrics programs. These are becoming part of the definition of good medical practice. But as valuable as these extensions are, they are still set in a medical care model, and they fall short of addressing concerns about and taking some responsibility for functional status, family caregivers, or access to formal community care services.

That story of innovation in an HMO is still here, but the issues that were encountered and the solutions that were tested are also relevant at a broader level. Aging, chronic illness, disability, and caregiving across the lifespan, and separation between medical and community care, are general issues both in the United States and around the world, and practical ways to connect with community care are very much needed.

According to conventional wisdom, expanding into community care is at once an obvious and a fool-hardy thing for an HMO to do. On the one hand, it seems obvious that an organization with the mission of maintaining and improving the health of its members would be concerned that its most vulnerable members may not be bathing or eating enough, or may not have transportation to the doctor; these are the types of needs that community care addresses. On the other hand, there are both imaginary and real problems that go along with trying to address these needs.

Two sets of questions need to be addressed when considering including community care in an integrated care delivery system, such as an HMO. The first set of questions addresses what an HMO should be doing to help get these services to HMO members, since most such services are provided by community organizations outside the span of influence of the medical care organization. Should it pay for services? Create them? Paying seems unlikely given the rising medical care costs for prescription drugs and other expensive technologies. And why duplicate what already exists through creating services? Thus the interest in integrating with organizations already delivering them through joint ventures, contracts, mergers.

It is not going to continue to be possible to ignore these issues, at least at the service delivery level. Deficits in in-home support of nutrition, transportation, socialization, and functioning not only can affect a health plan's ability to deliver on its primary medical care mission; they are legitimate concerns in themselves. Also of concern are members who are caregivers—do they know what they need to about caring for a loved-one with disabilities, are they overburdened, and do they know how to get help if they need it? As the numbers of people with disabilities living at home grows, these seem like ever more important concerns for an integrated health care delivery system.

On the other hand, the more important these issues become as service delivery matters, the more problematic they become on the benefits side. The common wisdom is that community care insurance is health care's tar baby—once you touch it you will get stuck with overwhelming demands for help. With women working more, and elders living longer, and children with disabilities living at home instead of in state institutions, overburdened caregivers are thought to be looking for a way out. The other metaphor is the woodwork effect: if you offer help people will come "out of the woodwork" to get it. Fearing the high costs and high demand, U.S. health insurers—both public and private—carefully guard the borders of their medical care coverage to define long-term supportive care as someone else's responsibility.

The competitive market in health insurance adds another reason not to insure community care needs. Even if a health plan's actual commitment to paying for new community care services is limited, just doing anything to raise its profile as a good place for the chronically ill or disabled seems suicidal from a market perspective. Even if you don't add costs directly, you're appealing to just the types of members that insurers don't want. In the last half of the 1990s and into the twenty-first century, the "smart money" in many health care markets has been cutting benefits that appeal to sick people (e.g., prescription drugs), and leaving market segments where large numbers of sick and disabled people are found (e.g., Medicare and Medicaid).

While it's tempting to go off on a tirade about the absurdity of the race to the bottom fostered by the market approach to insuring and delivering health care in the United States, that's not what this book is about. Rather, the intent is to examine and present the case for doing good and doing well in better serving members with disabilities. It is possible to reconcile the two sides of the dilemma posed above that is, to become a health care system that better understands and serves the community care needs of its at-risk members, that benefits from the improved supports in real ways, and that does not suffer from the increased costs or adverse selection of doing so. Drawing from the case examples of one HMO's demonstration of the outlines of such a model, the lessons are relevant to other HMOs and the health care system as a whole.

The separation of medical care and community care—and the careful guarding of the borders of medical care benefits—is also enshrined in the policies of the primary public payer in the U.S. health care system—Medicare. And it is common in definitions of health care benefits in most countries. Health insurance schemes do not appear to be ready to take on the costs or the service delivery responsibility of "long-term care," both for cost concerns and also out of concern that the "medical model" may not be the right solution for the variety of social and supportive services that comprise community care. As long as this is the case, the best practical solution may be to accept the formal separations and to develop models to make the two systems work better together. Those are the kinds of models that were developed and tested by KP.

But rather than getting ahead of the story, there is some groundwork to lay. Before health insurers and providers can take initiative in this area, there is a lot they need to know that they generally do not know about the community care system. This book reports on a model that was developed in an extraordinary KP demonstration program that counted heavily on forming collaborations with a wide range of community care agencies, volunteer resources, and family caregivers. Although the driving force in this initiative was an HMO, these community care resources provided much of the fuel to keep it going. These agencies and family members deserve a prominent place in the story, not just from the vantage of giving credit where credit is due, but also to provide lessons for other community care agencies, caregivers, and community care systems about how to work more closely and effectively with health care systems.

This first chapter, however, is primarily for acute care sector professionals, policy makers, and managers. It is designed to give needed background about community care missions, funding, programs, agencies, services, and clientele. That's a tall order, since the community care system is many overlapping systems covering numerous target groups from newborn babies to workers to very old retirees. And each of these systems at times hardly seems like a system at all, given the multiplicity of funders, targeting, and providers. The chapter cannot provide every detail, but it does give the broad outline of the system, and it highlights the themes that cut across the system for all age groups and types of disabilities. It also reviews prior efforts to better coordinate and even integrate the acute and long-term care sectors.

The chapter is written primarily—but not exclusively—from the point of view of U.S. experience and programs. However, some of the structural features of U.S. medical care and community care systems, as well as the professional and service delivery practices of the two systems, will resonate for non-U.S. readers, particularly in Europe and Canada. Most Western countries (and many others around the world) cover medical care as a universal entitlement through programs that are financed and regulated at the national level. In contrast, community care services are typically financed and organized at a local level, and most countries also impose some means testing for community care. The divisions in financing, coverage, and regulation parallel and foster professional and operational divisions between medical care and community care. The KP demonstration's approaches to overcoming these divisions are relevant to this broader audience.

This chapter's background on service systems is important not because it is necessary for every doctor and administrator to know everything about every community care service and agency in their community and how to use them; that would be a poor use of professional time, and it is not realistic to expect it will happen. But it is important to understand in general what community care agencies do, the types of clients they serve, the challenges they face, and what needs to happen for acute care and community care to work better together for mutual benefit. This chapter provides this picture of how community care services work and the good they can do for the people who use them.

Regrettably, there is not much hard, bottom-line evidence to present that the community care system saves money, or even if it does, that an HMO can capture any of the savings. Evidence is at best mixed from prior research and demonstrations, and the evidence from the KP demonstration is illustrative rather than definitive. Professionals, policy makers, and managers will need to judge for themselves whether there's enough evidence of value to move forward for broader and more definitive tests of coordinated medical/community care models.

DEMOGRAPHIC CHANGES AND CHANGING NEEDS

This section quickly reviews population data, to give a sense of which types of people may need help with community care, what their needs are, how numerous they are, and what kind of services would help. It's important to try to think beyond these data to try to see that disability, like illness, is just a part of peoples' lives. People are more than unmet needs to be matched with services, and providing services accomplishes more than just addressing needs.

Conceptions of Need

Most people with disabilities are aged, but the majority of aged people do not have significant disabilities. Public images of aging are prone to dueling stereotypes: fit and active retirees versus frail and dependent nursing home residents, socially engaged citizens versus lonely and homebound isolates, affluent globe-trotters versus impoverished residents of run-down senior housing, White and well-served versus Black and ill-served. Although such stereotypes are dangerous when applied to individuals, they do reflect the range of the realities of elders. The challenge for a health care system is to get beyond stereotyping and get to know and work with each elder as an individual.

In contrast to typical perception of elders, images of disabilities among working-age adults and children are perhaps less well formed. Since the closing of state institutions for the mentally and physically handicapped three decades ago, the advances in equal rights to education two decades ago, and the passage of the Americans with Disabilities Act 10 years ago, public awareness of the breadth of disability has grown, as have social obligations to create the conditions for the disabled to participate more fully in society.

Looking at the population as a whole (almost), nearly 49 million U.S. residents over age five (19.4%) have a disability of some type (Table 1.1). Of these, 24.1 million have a severe disability that requires the help of another person to perform an important activity. Of the noninstitutional population over age five, 4% (9.2 million persons) need personal assistance with one or more Activities of Daily Living (ADLs), including bathing, dressing, using the toilet, transferring from bed to chair, or eating, or an Instrumental ADL (IADL), including laundry, shopping, cleaning, cooking, money management, using the telephone, or taking medications. One percent (2.5 million) have a developmental disability or mental retardation.

For a large integrated health care system like Kaiser Permanente, which has more than 8 million members (including 800,000 Medicare members), these statistics translate into sobering figures: roughly 1.5 million members with some disability, 750,000 with a severe disability, 320,000 members needing help with ADLs, 80,000 with a developmental disability. Using a different measure of disability, one in seven of KP's members (560,000) are likely to have an activity limitation; of these, 180,000 are unable to perform a major activity—whether it be play, school, work, or personal care, depending on age.

The prevalence of most physical disabilities increases with age, while the prevalence of mental retardation and developmental disabilities is highest among those under age 18 (Krauss, Stoddard, & Gilmartin, 1996). Disability is closely tied to the number and severity of chronic illnesses (Cassel, Rudberg, & Olshansky, 1992; Guralnik et al., 1989), but even among elders, disability is often short-term, or at least characterized by ups and downs even though the long-term trajectory is toward greater impairment (Hallfors et al., 1994). Only 2% of those aged 65–69 need help from another person to perform ADLs, but this rises to 20% for those 85 and over. The prevalence of dementia rises from 2% to 30% for the same age groups. Since the fastest growing population segments are the oldest old, the proportions of the population with disabilities are projected to rise precipitously over the next decades.

Adding more variables puts a more personal face on the numbers. Because women live longer than men, there are about twice as many women over age 85 with a disability as there are men. And because women marry older men, most of these women are likely to be widows, who most often live alone. Although there are certainly rich widows, because women's pensions are on average much less than men's and because pensions and savings in general become less adequate at older ages, the prototypical elder with disabilities is female, widowed, living alone, and poor or near poor. These statistics vary some by race and ethnicity: African Americans acquire disabilities at younger ages but live shorter lives than whites. Asian Americans in general live longer.

TABLE 1.1   Numbers and Percentages of U.S. Population with Disabilities and Activity Limitations*

	Number	Percent of Population
Have a disability of some type (vision, hearing, talking, lifting 10 pounds, walking 1/4 mile, climbing stairs, mobility inside and outside the home, and getting in and out of bed)	49 million	19.4%
Have a severe disability (can't perform or needs help of another to perform any of the above)	24.1 million	9.6%
Need personal assistance with bathing, dressing, eating, transferring, or using the toilet or with an instrumental activity like shopping or cooking	9.2 million	4.0%
Have a developmental disability	2.5 million	1.0%
Have a limitation in performing a major activity, e.g., work, school, or play, depending on age	37.7 million	14.9%
Unable to perform major activity	12 million	4.8%

* Source: Krauss, Stoddard, & Gilmartin, 1996.

	Age 65–69	Age 85 & over
Need personal assistance with bathing, dressing, eating, transferring, or using the toilet	2%	20%

Source: LaPlante & Carlson, 1996.

Prevalence of dementia	2%	30%

Source: Small et al., 1997.

Another way to think about disability is a life-cycle perspective. People become disabled at different points in life—some from birth, some in midlife, and others not until old age. Timing affects what persons have been able to do before they became disabled, including following typical work and family patterns, which can create the financial and social assets that help many face disability in old age. The timing of disablement also affects preferences and expectations. School-age and working-age persons with disabilities prioritize supports that help them maintain age-appropriate social roles—for example, going to school and working, respectively. Age-appropriate social roles are different for those who become disabled in old age, but nonetheless important to them. On another level, impairments that foster disabilities are of different types, intensities, and trajectories. The impact of a short-term disability from which a person recovers is different from a short-term degenerative disability, which is in turn different from a long-term stable disability.

Caregivers

About three-quarters of the help provided to persons with disabilities is given by "informal" caregivers—that is, family members, close friends, and neighbors. Fears about the woodwork effect notwithstanding, these caregivers help not just because there is no alternative formal help available. Rather, for a wide variety of reasons, both caregivers and care receivers prefer it that way. This is not to say that caregivers don't want or use help from formal systems when it is available, just that there is not much evidence that formal help is overused or abused. Rather, it appears that people substitute formal services for informal selectively—for example, adding case management to get the things that case managers most easily control (personal care and homemakers), substituting when a caregiver is lost because of death or illness, and substituting temporarily during periods of increased need (Tennstedt, Crawford, & McKinlay, 1993).

While studies have described the positive effects of caregiving to frail and older family members (Farran, 1997; Fredman, Daly, & Lazur, 1995, Archbold et al., 1992), caregiving has also been linked to stress and role strain (Anthony, Zarit, & Gatz, 1998; Archbold et al., 1990; Deimling & Bass, 1986; Emanuel et al., 2000; Levine, 1999), as well as to negative health outcomes (Archbold, 1982; Coppel et al., 1985). The risk appears to be greatest for overburdened spouses; in one study, older spouses who were caregivers and experiencing strain were 63% more likely to die over a four-year study period than controls, after controlling for sociodemographics and prevalent disease (Schulz & Beach, 1999). Caregiving has also been shown to increase vulnerability to flu, low immune function, and depression. Again, spousal caregivers are particularly vulnerable: even though in general married persons are healthier than the unmarried, this changes when the spouse gets ill (Kiecolt-Glaser & Glaser, 1999).

Studies of caregiving reveal several patterns of caring, some of which appear to be riskier than others (Twigg & Atkin, 1994). One risky pattern is restrictiveness—i.e., the notion that caregivers' movements are restricted by their roles, in part because of anxiety about what could happen in their absence. Others (mostly females) become "engulfed" by caring—i.e., obscured by the person for whom they are caring. But still other caregivers are able to balance and maintain boundaries. These caregivers are more assertive, have a stronger sense of deserving help, and are easier to involve in a problem-solving approach. Yet others reach a symbiosis with the cared-for person, which is defined as derived outside of marriage. This relationship causes fewer problems for the caregiver.

Mixing caring and working brings its own risks, including fewer hours of care provided when caregivers work more hours (Doty, Jackson, & Crown, 1998). Women have been found to reduce hours to meet caregiving demands, leading to economic disadvantage (Pavalko & Artis, 1997). Unlike the practice in some European countries (Evers, 1995), disability and retirement benefits are not available in the United States on the basis of providing family care to a family member with disabilities. Finally, it is difficult to overemphasize the fact that caring and its consequences are primarily the domain of women—mothers, daughters, and spouses (Baldwin & Twigg, 1991; Barnes & Walker, 1996; England et al., 1991; Farkas & Himes, 1997; Harrington, 1998; Walker, 1984). Caregiver support and training is just a part of a much larger package of supports needed to compensate for the unequal burdens faced by women caregivers (Twigg & Atkin, 1994).

The life cycle concept also helps untangle the relative stresses and burdens of caregiving. For example, for the first year or two of life, a child with a physical impairment causing lower body paralysis may require the same care as a typically developing infant, and society considers it normal that parents (particularly mothers) provide this care as a matter of course. As the children age, however, their care needs will increase—eventually to the point where they will be too heavy for the mother to lift and where (if the child is male), sexual taboos may interfere with her ability to help with toileting, dressing, and bathing (Litwak, Jessop, & Moulton, 1994). Also, the teen turning 20 will want a life independent of his parents. These are very different family care relationships than those of a wife's caring for her husband of 50 years. Similarly, the aged caregiving wife is in a different life-cycle point than a daughter/career of working age, and may expect different help from the community care system (Gerry & Mirsky, 1992).

THE RESPONSE TO NEED

This section reviews the types of help that may be available in a particular community and who pays for that help. The term "may" is used because effective access to community care varies tremendously by age, type of disability, level of disability, income and assets, and geography. In contrast to acute care, community care is for the most part not an entitlement. Funding and access are predetermined rather than need- or demand-driven. Unfortunately, the predetermined levels are too often inadequate.

The community care system also responds to needs related to chronic illness and disability in different ways than does the acute/medical care system. Whereas the latter provides cures, prevention, and rehabilitation, the former for the most part provides support, substitution, and amelioration. The medical care system is also more unified as a delivery system; its professionals are of higher status and its finances are much more ample and secure.

Services

Before moving into the complexity of the system of financing and delivering care, let's just look at the basic things that are provided. Community care encompasses a wide range of services (e.g., homemakers, personal care aides, transportation, adult day care) for people who need help related to activities of daily living such as bathing, dressing and using the toilet, instrumental activities such as shopping, cleaning, and cooking, as well as incontinence, mobility, and transportation. Care also addresses need for supervision due to cognitive impairment—perhaps to keep a person from wandering off or perhaps to help arrange medications. Care can be direct hands-on help from an aide, or it can be in the form of supplies or equipment, such as walkers, grab bars, bath benches, and personal emergency response systems which can be activated to call for help if a person falls and cannot get up. Working-age people with disabilities may have additional services—for example, vocational rehabilitation and training in independent living—while school-age children with disabilities will likely receive educational supports and newborns and preschoolers with developmental delays or established risks like cerebral palsy or Down Syndrome may receive enrichment, therapies, or family support. Finally, the system may provide a case manager or care coordinator, who can help the individual or family to figure out what they need, facilitate access to public financing, and organize the provision of help. Because most of community care takes place in the home, community care providers and case managers become involved in the complexity of personal and family relationships (Fischer & Eustis, 1994).

Community Care Versus Skilled Home Health Care

For many people the first contact with in-home support is with the kind of services covered under Medicare's skilled home health benefit, and many of the community care services described above could be delivered through medical care insurance of skilled home health. But there are crucial differences. To qualify for Medicare coverage, patients must be homebound, under the care of a physician, require the care of a "skilled" nurse or therapist, and be recovering from an acute condition (Bishop & Skwara, 1993).[1] When these conditions are met, home health is covered as an entitlement for most Americans, and a great deal of help with ADLs can be provided as collateral services by home health aides. But there are catches, and these form the pathways into the need for community care.

---

[1] Private health insurance coverage is structured in similar ways, and HMOs like KP generally follow the coverage practices of Medicare and other private insurers in authorizing skilled home health services. Medical care systems in other countries also make these kinds of distinctions in order to draw the lines between where they end and community care systems pick up.

One catch is that even while receiving Medicare-covered home health care, many patients have unmet community care needs. One study of 2,013 home health patients selected to represent visits for Acquired-Immune Deficiency Syndrome (AIDS), hospice, intravenous therapy, and more common types of visits found unmet need (among those with need) as follows: homemaker (39%), home health aide (28%), equipment (9%), mental health (56%), social work (45%), transport (30%), occupational therapy (36%), speech therapy (51%), and nutrition (25%). Focus groups with nurses attributed unmet need to non-reimbursable services, lack of supply, physicians' orders not matching their patients' needs, and hospital discharge planners' not arranging the correct mix of support services (Thomas & Payne, 1998). Even the home health directors working within HMOs are so influenced by their peers in the home health field that they continue to view the world through fee-for-service glasses (Greenlick & Brody, 1997).

Another shortcoming is that most people don't improve in ability to perform ADLs before Medicare coverage runs out, and more than 20% are not even stabilized at discharge (Shaughnessy et al., 1996). Often the nurse's expectations and the reality of the informal support structure are incongruent, including the difficulties of scheduling visits to teach the family members what they need to know to maintain or improve the patient's functioning. A third shortcoming is that only a quarter to a third of the Medicare population with ADL dependencies ever meet skilled care criteria in the course of a year (Mauser, 1997; Williams & Weissert, 1994). Finally, the 1997 Balanced Budget Act (BBA) reduced even these levels of service to long-term patients by creating incentives for agencies to discharge high-visit patients (Komisar & Feder, 1998; Liu, Wissoker, & Rimes, 1998).[2]

Once entitled skilled care benefits run out, patients enter the long-term care system, and virtually everything changes. First, at least when it comes to in-home support, service providers tend to be paraprofessionals—e.g., homemakers, personal care attendants. Second, access based on medical status as determined by physicians is replaced by access based on functional status, usually determined by nurses or social workers, or in the case of children, by developmental status as determined by educators, psychologists, and therapists. Third, for most supports in the home and community for adults, entitlement is replaced by private pay, means testing, and public programs that are too sparsely funded to meet demand.[3] Fourth, whereas medical care is

---

[2] The BBA did through payment reform what had been difficult to do through changes in eligibility regulations without court interference, i.e., cut off long-term home health users. Under the BBA, eligibility for care plan management and evaluation remains a "skilled" service for beneficiaries with complex conditions, and the home health aides continue to be a covered collateral service. It's just that prospective payment for long-term cases no longer covers costs. Thus agencies rather than intermediaries and the federal government are the ones limiting service.

[3] Many children's services are an exception, especially entitled educational services.

typically paid by a unitary source, community care services are paid by a wide range of public and private sources. Fifth, along with institutional long-term care, paraprofessional community care agencies face a staffing crisis fueled by the low wages, poor training, and inadequate supervision that many such agencies suffer because of inadequate reimbursement. This makes it difficult to find agencies with adequate staff who are reliable and knowledgeable. And finally, when caregivers and patients move to long-term care, they feel the shift in the way they are treated personally by medical and nursing professionals, who heap attention and care during the acute phase of care but who may lose interest and understanding when it becomes the caregiver's responsibility to create necessary supports in the community (Cooley, 1992; Levine, 1999). In one Canadian study of eight caregivers for post-traumatic brain injury patients, in the whole course of setting up care after rehabilitation, none of the eight caregivers found a professional who would say they were responsible (Smith & Smith, 2000).

Medicaid Coverage of Community Care Services

These problems exist even for the population with the strongest entitlement to community care services: Medicaid eligibles. A common misconception is that the poor are covered for community care through Medicaid. In fact, nursing facility care is Medicaid's only mandatory long-term care service; states are not required to offer community care services beyond skilled home health.

Most states, however, do cover some community care through Medicaid, either as "optional" services or "waiver" services. Optional services include personal care, case management, and adult day care. If a state chooses to offer an optional service, it must make it available statewide to all Medicaid beneficiaries who meet eligibility criteria. Some states use the personal care benefit to fund personal care attendants, which is a core service in the independent living model for working-age adults with disabilities. Other states use personal care attendants extensively for elders (Rodat, Griesbach, & Zadoorian, 1997).

To target Medicaid community care services more narrowly and/or to enrich the package of services, states can ask for waivers of amount, duration, and scope of Medicaid services. The only accepted policy rationale for states to request waivers and for the federal government to grant them is that community care is keeping beneficiaries out of more expensive nursing homes. By late 1996, there were more than 220 community care waiver programs in existence in all states (Mitchell, 1996). Waivers allow states to create a tailored package of services (e.g., a long list of community care supports or a particular one like group homes), that will be targeted toward a particular group (e.g., elders, developmentally disabled), and that perhaps will be available only in particular locales, and only for a designated number of beneficiaries at one time. Restrictions also apply to the most disabled: Some state community care programs exclude the most dependent because their needs cannot be met within program spending limits (Liu, Hanson, & Coughlin, 1995). Waiting lists can be established for waivered services, and historically they have often been long.

Long waiting lists were one factor of the 1990 Olmstead v. L. C. et al. decision by the Supreme Court that ruled on the basis of the Americans with Disabilities Act that two institutionalized persons with mental disabilities had a right to community care since others equally disabled were living in community settings (Rosenbaum, 2000). The ruling applies not just to the institutionalized who would like to be in community, but also to those in the community who would like an institution, and those in the community who would like community care support but are not getting it. The implications of the Olmstead decision will take years to play out in actual access to community care services.

Other Community Care Service

While Medicaid is the major single funder of long-term care services, both in the community and institutions, a plethora of smaller programs funded by the federal, state, and local governments round out the community care system of care (Wiener & Sullivan, 1995). These are generally targeted at particular age groups, disabilities, or types of service, and it is not possible to even mention them all here. Highlights start with the youngest, including the Department of Education's Early Intervention program, which provides family support, therapies, and developmental support for children with disabilities from birth to age three. Babies, children, and adults may also be eligible for condition-related support from state departments of mental retardation. At age three, school systems pick up much of the responsibility for broadly defined educational supports, with a variety of state and federal funding support. After school age (18–21), some young adults are able to continue getting support from the vocational rehabilitation/education systems.

Another source of support for both younger and older persons with severe disabilities is Supplemental Security Income (SSI). SSI not only provides a small income, but also carries with it eligibility for Medicaid, which is the key for access not only to medical care benefits but also to Medicaid personal care and waiver services. Waivers allow Medicaid to pay for group homes, transportation, and in-home support to family caregivers. Finally, most states supplement SSI with a housing allowance that supports many adults with a variety of physical and mental disabilities in board and care homes, group homes, and assisted living.

Working age people who become disabled are eligible for Social Security Disability Insurance (SSDI) if they have just a few quarters of covered employment. The level of income from SSDI is tied to employment history, but any level brings Medicare eligibility. While this structure of income, health, and long-term care benefits is helpful, both SSI and SSDI income and service benefits are lost when beneficiaries work. This is one reason that persons with disabilities generally have very low incomes (Davis & O'Brien, 1996).

Besides being available via these entitlement-based benefit systems (health insurance, Medicare, Medicaid, SSI, education), community care is generally offered through service programs. Whereas "entitled benefits" implies access to a set of covered services on an equitable basis for a defined group of eligible individuals, a service program can offer limited types or amounts of services, establish waiting lists, and make no pretense of meeting either an individual's or a population's actual need or demands.

The best example of a service program in the community care services field is the aging networks supported by the Older Americans Act (OAA).[4] The aging network is administered by the federal Administration on Aging and 57 designated State Units on Aging (including the District of Columbia and U.S. Territories), which in turn support 650 Area Agencies on Aging (AAAs) across the country.[5] The AAAs are the hub for the system, and OAA-funded community care services include supportive in-home and community-based services, congregate and home-delivered meals, transportation, senior centers, health promotion, a new caregiver support program, homemaker services, and information and referral. Priority for direct services is for lower income elders age 60 and older.

The network has a reasonable administrative and service shell, but the OAA provides only limited funding to keep it going ($1.1 billion in FY 2002 for the entire OAA), with less than half for direct community care services for frail elders and their caregivers (OAA, 2001). Many states supplement the funding and power of AAAs by giving them control of additional funds for community care services from state general revenues, the federal Social Services Block Grant, and Medicaid community care waivers. Some other states consolidate funding and case management in state or county agencies (Leutz et al., 1992).

However, even in the relatively consolidated and well-funded states, community care programs fall well short of providing an entitlement to

---

[4] An analog to the OAA and the aging network for working-age persons with disabilities are the network of Centers for Independent Living (CILs), which are funded by the federal Rehabilitation Act and administered by state departments of rehabilitation. Their core services have traditionally been peer counseling, independent living skills training, information and referral, and advocacy. In a few states, they have taken on some role in providing or arranging direct services, e.g., personal care attendants.

[5] In some states, the State Unit works statewide and there are no AAAs.

community care for all frail elders, or even for low-income elders. Those who are most disabled seldom can be kept in the community without family care (Abrahams et al., 1989; Long, 1995). In the most poorly funded states, in-home support for ADLs and IADLs is hard to get, expensive, and of poor quality in many communities (Rabiner et al., 1997). Fortunately for the KP demonstration, the states in which most of the projects took place (CA, OR, WA, HI, CO) are among those with stronger aging networks (Leutz et al., 1992).

In summary, because community care services are optional state benefits under Medicaid, and because numerous smaller community care service programs aim at particular groups of persons with disabilities, differences occur both across and within states in which groups receive public support, how much they receive, and under what conditions (Leutz et al., 1992; Liu, Hanson, & Coughlin, 1995). The result is a system of "haves" and "have nots," with some people stuck in "no care zones" in which their age, disability status, location, or income exclude them from assistance which they formerly had or which others with no greater apparent need seem to enjoy (Kassner & Martin, 1996; Litvak & Kennedy, 1991).

The uneven nature of public coverage for long-term care in both institutions and the community has caused many to look to the private sector to solve the problem. Even with help from foundations and tax subsidies to jump-start the private market, the private sector has not yet come close to solving the social problem of financing long-term care. The number of long-term care insurance policies sold is increasing (perhaps 10% of elders have bought policies), but policies are affordable only to the well-off (Crown, Burwell, & Alecxih, 1994; McCall, Bauer, & Korb, 1996; Rivlin & Wiener, 1988). Also, statistics about the number of policies sold are misleading, since insurers report that half of the policies they sell will lapse in five years and that 65% will lapse in 10 years (GAO, 1993). In recent years insurers have improved products with the addition of community care coverage and contracts with care coordination agencies, but these additions have not changed the market, which is incapable of reaching those most in need today—middle to low-income persons and those who already have chronic illnesses and disabilities. Thus long-term insurance basically serves an estate-protection function and does little to finance needed long-term care services.

Finally, a discussion of the community-based resources available to help people with disabilities and their caregivers would not be complete without mention of national and local voluntary and self-help organizations. These include large organizations such as the Alzheimer's and Related Disorders Association, the Stroke Association, United Cerebral Palsy, and the Multiple Sclerosis Society, as well as smaller volunteer efforts organized by churches, fraternal organizations, businesses, health care providers, and neighborhood groups. These and other organizations support information and referral lines, support groups, direct services such as adult day care, and service coordination. They are supported by endowments, volunteers, tax deductible donations, auctions, walkathons, raffles, and the like. KP itself has a community benefit fund paid for by small monthly additions to member premiums, as well as a community giving fund supported by voluntary contributions of employees. Because these voluntary and self-help organizations are often staffed by persons who use services themselves, help seekers can get first-hand information that is relevant to local areas. Their simple acts of help such as friendly visiting, shopping, and transportation to social events can fill key gaps in the formal system, and they fill those gaps in very a personalized and caring manner.

Spending on Community Care Services

Service users, families, and policy makers tend to prefer home care to institutional long-term care, but the bulk of public long-term care funds are spent on nursing facilities. In fiscal year 1999, spending on long-term care by Medicaid was $62.4 billion, including $36.4 billion (58%) on nursing facilities, $9.6 billion (16%) on institutional care for persons with mental retardation, and $16.4 billion (26%) on home-based and community-based services, including home health, personal care, and home- and community-based waiver services (Doty, 2000).

Looking at spending for elders only, Table 1.2 shows that an even higher portion of Medicaid funds for elders goes to institutional care (86%). Medicare was the biggest public spender on home care, but, as was shown above, this primarily covered skilled services rather than long-term community care, and services to the longer-term patients that fueled the rise in Medicare home health spending in the 1990s were cut way back by the 1997 BBA (Bishop, Kerwin, & Wallack, 1999; OIG, 1999; Stone, 2000; Welch, Wennberg, & Welch, 1996). Other public funders of community care services do not make up for the lack of Medicare coverage of long-term home care, or the focus of Medicaid funds on the very poor (AARP, 1995; Alecxih, Corea, & Kennell, 1995; Pepper Commission, 1990; Wiener & Sullivan, 1995). In 1995, other state and federal spending on community care services for elders amounted only to $2.1 billion (Committee on Ways & Means, 1996). Private out-of-pocket spending was the biggest source of spending on long-term home care.

Looking at spending on a per capita basis, Table 1.3 shows that in 1995 Medicaid spent more than $1,000 per year on community care services per Medicaid-eligible elder living in the community (i.e., not in a nursing home). This reflects the relatively high rates of disability among Medicaid eligibles and also the relatively generous benefits in Medicaid compared to Medicare and private insurance coverage. On average, non-Medicaid elders spent about one-sixth this much of their own money on community care. All other

TABLE 1.2   Spending by (for) Elders by Source: NH/HC 1995 (Billions)

	Nursing Facility	Home and Community	Total
Medicare	$5.5	$9.4	$14.9
Medicaid	$23.5	$3.8	$27.3
Other Federal	$0.7	$1.6	$2.3
Other state and local	$0.6	$0.5	$1.1
Out of pocket	$28.2	$5.2	$33.4
Private insurance	$0.1	$0.1	$0.2
	$58.6	$20.6	$79.2

An unknown portion of $2.8 billion in Social Services Block Grant funds in 1996 was allocated to HCB services for elders.

Source: Committee on Ways and Means (1996). *The green book* (Table TB-11). Washington, DC: U.S. House of Representatives.

federal community care service funding for elders in general was barely $4 per person per month. Given that about one in 10 elders has a disability that might require personal care, this level of funding would be enough to pay for, at most, two visits a month per frail elder. This is perhaps enough visits for homemaker service, but it is completely inadequate for a person who needs daily personal care. Other state and local spending was not even a third of these other federal funds, and private insurance was a trivial source on a per capita basis, reflecting the very low penetration of long-term care insurance policies.

In conclusion, while the sources of public funding for community care services are inadequate and that many individuals do not have the resources to pay for adequate services out-of-pocket, there are community care resources in most communities that are worth tapping. Some people with disabilities and their families can pay directly. A few can qualify for a strong public package. Many others are between these two poles and may qualify for a few gap-filling services and find some volunteer assistance to help out families, who provide most of the care.

RATIONALES FOR INCREASING SUPPORT FOR COMMUNITY CARE SERVICES

So what is it that holds back spending on community care services? The general answer goes back in part to English and American Poor Law traditions of aversion to outdoor versus indoor relief (Holstein & Cole, 1996). Fearing that poor, old, and disabled people would take advantage of public support

TABLE 1.3 Per Capita Spending on In-home and Community-based Long-Term Care Services by Source (1995)

	Annual	Monthly
US Medicaid HCB spending per Medicaid community elder	$1,031	$85.91
US private out-of pocket spending/non-Medicaid community elder	$161	$13.44
US Other federal spending/non-Medicaid community elder	$50	$4.14
Other state and local/non-Medicaid community elder	$16	$1.29
Private insurance spending per non-Medicaid community elder	$3	$0.26

Sources:
Numbers of Medicaid-eligible and non-Medicaid elders: AARP (1998)

Across the states: Profiles of long-term care systems. Washington, DC: Public Policy Institute, and AARP (1997). Reforming the health care system: state profiles 1997. Washington, DC: Public Policy Institute.

Community spending data from: Committee on Ways and Means. (1996) The Green Book. Washington, DC: US House of Representatives.

in the comfort of their homes, towns and states tended to use the rigors of the poorhouse to separate the "truly needy" from those who could get by on their own or with help from their families. In the 19th and well into the 20th century, local poorhouses were increasingly supplanted by state hospitals for the mentally and physically disabled. And these in turn gave way to Medicaid-funded institutions (nursing homes and intermediate care facilities for the mentally retarded [ICF/MRs]) after federal support for care and income for people with disabilities became available through Medicaid and SSI in the 1960s and 1970s.

Policy debates over increasing public support for community care services as alternatives to institutions have continued to be influenced by these same themes: the fear of supplanting family responsibility, questions about the relative costs of institutional versus community-based service alternatives, and working through which levels of government should shoulder costs (and realize savings) of alternative approaches.

Additionally, however, questions about outcomes for those who use the community-based service system have gained importance, and they have been tested in a series of demonstrations over the last several decades. These include improved health outcomes, intrinsic benefits to users, and supporting caregivers. Some of these rationales could also justify investment in community care services by the medical care system. The search for a rationale for moving forward with the KP demonstration model thus fits in a longer search for meaning and value in community care. Unfortunately, most of these outcomes have been difficult to document, and this has led both to disappointment, periodic rethinking and repackaging of rationales, and calls for more high-profile research and policy analysis (Callahan, 2000).

Efficiency

The most compelling rationale for expanding community care has been achieving savings through the efficiency of substituting lower-cost community care services for more expensive ones, particularly to reduce nursing home and hospital care for elders and as alternatives to state institutions for younger persons with physical and developmental disabilities. Home care was sold as a service that would pay for itself through substituting for care in these other, less desirable settings. While this seemed plausible in the days of long hospital stays and intermediate care nursing homes, net savings proved hard to achieve, even though some programs did reduce the use of these other services (Kemper, Applebaum, & Harrigan, 1987; Weissert & Cready, 1989).

As the acuity and dependency levels of patients in institutional care have risen in intervening years, the idea that community care can be a widespread alternative is increasingly implausible. In the few specific cases where programs have saved money through substitutions, or where comprehensive models have survived, they have done it by carefully targeting a specific segment of the frail population (e.g., post-acute patients [Smith et al., 1988], nursing home applicants [Blackman, Brown, & Leaner, 1986], Medicaid eligibles [Laudicina & Burwell, 1988; Eggert et al., 1991], persons with Alzheimer's Disease [Newcomer et al., 1999], or the wealthy [Crown, Capitman, & Leutz 1992; Rivlin & Wiener, 1988]). They succeeded on this basis, but they thereby excluded the much larger number of individuals who were in fact disabled but did not fit or who did not want the approach offered. Broader targeting on the basis of need as measured by functional status was found to increase net costs, because it brought services to people who would not have used nursing home or hospital care in the absence of formal community care services. Whether or not the expansion of the number of users was evidence of a "woodwork effect," it has proven difficult to achieve net savings when services are provided to people who simply need help because they are disabled but who would probably not have gone into a nursing home without the service. Thus, an HMO looking for savings in acute care may find it in improving its post-acute services, but it is unlikely to find it in a broad-based expansion of community care services.

Outcomes

Another early rationale for spending more money on community care services was to improve outcomes, both hard outcomes such as slowing the rate of functional decline or lowering mortality and morbidity, and softer outcomes such as increasing users' sense of security and satisfaction or strengthening caregivers. Like cost savings, hard outcomes have been difficult to achieve, except when related to traditional medical system services—e.g., occupational therapy for frail elders (Clark et al., 1997), or use of advanced practice nurses for post-acute care (Naylor et al., 1999). However, there have been rather consistent successes with the soft outcomes such as satisfaction, sense of security, and decreases in caregiver burden (Newcomer et al., 1999; Weissert & Cready, 1989; Yordi, 1991). There may be benefits to the medical system from these effects, but they have been difficult to document directly.

Another type of intrinsic rationale relates to community care services as the means to achieving independence, choice, and autonomy for people with disabilities. These goals were framed by advocates of younger people with disabilities—including parents of children with disabilities and working-age adults with disabilities—and they were aimed at the dominant mode of community care—the so-called medical model of case management and purchased services. These were critiqued as not only wasteful but alienating, and an independent living model with a personal attendant hired, trained, and supervised by service users was advocated (Batavia, DeJong, & McKnew, 1991). Dependency-related and illness-related terms such as "client" and "patient" were disparaged in favor of "consumers" and "customers."

In recent years, the logical conclusion of the consumer model—cash for services—has been advocated and tried in the United States and abroad. It has a wide array of advocates (Doty, Matthias, & Franke, 1999; NCOA, 1997), as well as others who question whether everyone wants these responsibilities (Barnes & Prior, 1996; Capitman & Sciegaj, 1995; Simon-Rusinowitz et al., 1997) and whether the market can really deliver (Evers, Pijl, & Ungerson, 1994; Leutz, 1998). But even if one does not embrace cash as the solution to all community care service problems, it is clear that traditional case management/purchase of service approaches could do a better job of hearing peoples' preferences and incorporating them into care planning (Leutz, Sciegaj, & Capitman, 1997). Since people with disabilities have been in the forefront of the consumer choice movement in health care, there may be both direct and indirect benefits to a health care system that embraces working with advocates and patient groups around empowerment and autonomy issues.

INTEGRATION OF MEDICAL AND COMMUNITY CARE SYSTEMS

At the heart of the rationale for the Manifesto 2005 demonstration is the need to more closely connect medical care and community care, and at the heart of medical/community care connection initiatives is the concept of "integration." In the 1990s integration became a health policy mantra as an antidote to the fragmentation of care systems, but it was a mantra that has had different meanings to different people. Integration comes in degrees— running from "full integration," in which financing and delivery of a broad ranges of services is combined into a single organization, to "coordination," and "linkage," which connect the systems through less formalized communication, referral, educational, and care management arrangements.

The rationales for integration hark back to the original community care demonstration goals—system savings and improved outcomes. But integration is put forward as a much stronger model for achieving these goals than the early approach of simply adding community care services to the system (Capitman, Abrahams, & MacAdam, 1990; Greene, Ondrich, & Laditka, 1998; Wiener & Skaggs, 1995), since integrated systems are perceived to have incentives to use cheaper and appropriate community care services when they can substitute for expensive medical services.

Of course, before there was the idea of integrating medical and community care, there was integration of acute care itself in HMOs, as well as proposals to integrate community care services. Examples of the latter include pooling funds and control of all long-term care in Local Area Management Organization (Ruchlin, Morris, & Eggert, 1982), and creating community care management organizations to control Medicare post-acute care and community long-term care (Leutz et al., 1992). More recently, integration has been used to describe efforts to consolidate sub-parts of medical care (e.g., hospital care and post-acute rehab). The Clinton Health Plan proposal to have all Americans join managed care stimulated widespread integration of acute care sectors, and also spawned research that questioned whether managed care did a good job caring for persons with chronic illnesses or disabilities (Coleman et al., 2000; Retchin et al., 1992; Schnelle et al., 1999; Yelin, Lindsey, & Feigenbaum, 1996) or a bad job (Batavia 1993; Morgan et al., 1997; Schlenker, Shaughnessy, & Hittle, 1995; Shaughnessy, Schlenker, & Hittle, 1994; Ware et al., 1996). Answering these questions was part of the motivation behind broader integration efforts.

Many believe that the ideal model for integration of medical and community/long-term care is a managed care organization that is paid on a per capita basis for both acute and long-term care and that takes responsibility for delivering the whole range of services. The hypothesis is that integration aligns the incentives within a single organization, and it no longer matters whether it is Medicare or Medicaid that benefits from downward substitution or an emphasis on prevention. The benefits now go to the organization and beneficiaries, with benefits to payers accruing in eventual discounts on their capitations. These seem like win-win-win propositions for HMOs, payers, and beneficiaries.

"Laws" of Integration

Despite these conceptual advantages, integration has been very difficult to pull off in reality, as shall be seen presently. Leutz (1999) studied U.S. and U.K. integration initiatives and came up with five simple "laws" that help explain why. Perhaps the most important is, "You can't integrate a square peg in a round hole." This law stems from all the differences between medical care and community care that have been reviewed earlier in this chapter. Medical and community care are supported by different payers and bureaucracies. They operate on entitlement versus means testing, diagnosis and disease versus functional status, cure versus care, services primarily delivered by professionals versus paraprofessionals and family members, adequate national and employer funding versus inadequate state and local and individual funding. The financing differences are the most problematic: how can you integrate medical and community care funding when the streams of funding for the latter are so uneven? The large majority of the population are paying out-of-pocket for community care, a minority are eligible for welfare-based funding, and other parts of the public system are controlled by waiting lists and other artificial limits on supply.

The answer to these dilemmas about medical and community care differences is a second law of integration: "You can integrate all of the services for some of the people, some of the services for all of the people, but you can't integrate all of the services for all of the people." This law refers to the fact that there are different degrees to which medical and community care systems can be integrated, and it posits that one need not try to integrate in the same ways for everyone. Rather, three broad levels of integration can be described—linkage, coordination, and full integration—each in turn more appropriate for individuals with different types of needs in relation to severity, stability, duration, urgency, scope of services, and capacity for self-direction. Operationally, the three integration levels vary by degree of pooling of funds, creation of new community care support benefits, screening for those in need, coordination of clinical practice, case management, and information sharing. Each type of integration can be present alone or in combination in the same larger system.

A "fully integrated" system pools financing from medical, community care, and perhaps institutional long-term care payers; creates new types of benefits offered by the contracted, at-risk provider organization; and creates interdisciplinary teams to manage participants' access to the new benefits. Full integration is most appropriate for individuals with complex and unstable conditions and long-term social support needs that may encompass several and changing services.

A "coordinated" system uses case managers rather than teams to coordinate care, and the goal is to better manage access to existing services. Procedures are established between medical and community care providers to identify potential users at key points (e.g., discharge planning), to share information routinely across systems, and to manage the borders of coverage so that users have smooth transitions and maximum use of benefits. Coordination is appropriate for individuals with more stable conditions and relatively routine service needs that may be either short-term or long-term.

A "linked" system uses population screening to identify emergent community care needs and then refers those identified to existing services based on a good understanding of the targeting and goals of those services. There is no cross-system care management or planned information sharing, although information is provided when requested. To initiate linkage, medical care systems need to understand who pays for what and is eligible for what in community care, and to have staff who can make appropriate referrals to community care agencies and follow up on those referrals. Linkage can help empower people with mild to moderate disabilities that are self-directed to find specific services for routine needs of a short-term or long-term nature.

In summary, linkage and coordination generally take medical and social care systems as they are and try to make them work better together. They do not require waivers, contracts, multidisciplinary teams, or financing new benefits. But they do require medical and social systems to do something that they seldom do now—i.e., work together on a personal, real time basis around helping individuals served in both systems. Both linkage and coordination require clinicians—including physicians—to talk about disability and social care with their patients. Most of the onus for action rests with the medical system, but there are also things social care can do, not the least important of which is to expand and improve the community care system itself. As will be shown in the chapters that follow, the linkage and coordination concepts proved to be valuable guides for developing, implementing, and analyzing the Manifesto 2005 demonstration.

Three other "laws of integration" deserve mention before turning to a discussion of real-world examples. One is "Integration costs before it pays." This is clear to anyone who has ever tried to integrate services, but it's not always clear to policy makers or program administrators who are looking for quick savings from the efficiencies that would-be integrators promise. And the costs are not just planning money or new staff for the new coordination teams. It also should include new service money to sweeten the pot for the providers and agencies you are trying to integrate. Without new service resources, it can easily look like "you" are trying to get "me" to do "your" job with resources that are insufficient to do the job "I" already have.

Another law is "Your integration is my fragmentation." The drive for integration comes from professionals who are involved with a particular group that "needs" integrated services: poor and frail elders, infants with developmental delays, teens with physical disabilities making the transition from school to work, etc. The would-be integrator's focus is on how quality, efficiency, access, user control, and the like break down as a person needs help from multiple professionals and systems. So they ask professionals and managers in these systems to work together. The problem comes when professionals and managers get similar requests from many different groups. Particularly in the case of physicians—key players in most integration models—integration can be experienced as fragmentation—or as one group of U.K. physicians called it, "consultation fatigue" (Glendinning & Lloyd, 1997). Would-be integrators need to be sensitive to other demands on providers and consider carefully what level of participation to expect.

The final law is "The one who integrates calls the tune." This is related to "Your integration is my fragmentation" in that it acknowledges that everyone approaches integration with his/her own view of how to improve coordination of care for the disabled. If one wants to solve a particular coordination problem, one had better empower an individual to lead the effort that subscribes to that problem. Medical care providers tend to see discontinuities within the medical system, while practitioners within community care may see discontinuities there. They may not be the people to empower if the issue is better coordination across these two systems. So the lesson for policy makers and managers is to give the integration job to someone who wants to solve the problem that you want to solve.

Roles for Service Users

Where do service users fit when it comes to "calling the tune"? Effective inclusion at the policy and program design level takes support for the process and sensitivity to special needs, including thinking through how to gain fair representation (Bewley & Glendinning, 1994), setting meetings at times and places that are convenient, offering help with transportation and communications, putting in the staff and other resources that are required, and ensuring that the wishes of service users and families are heard and honored. The Interagency Coordinating Council form used to oversee federal Title 5 education funds for early intervention is a good example. It includes hiring parents of children with disabilities in designated staff positions in state government, and parents and providers meet publicly and regularly to consider and advise on policy and program.

Care needs to be taken that participatory processes are inclusive, since they can go wrong too—for example, through a tyranny of majority or domination by the articulate middle class (Barton, 1993). Consumerism is an individualist notion—maximizing one's own needs and satisfaction without reference to others with similar needs. Empowerment of one person should not result in disempowerment of another (Barnes & Walker, 1996). The process should ensure that all interests are represented fairly.

Participation of service users implies changes in procedures, power relationships, status, and security for professionals, who have investment and experience in running the system (Schorr, 1992). Service users are conditioned to deferring to professionals or at least telling them what they seem to want to hear (Clark, Dyer, & Hartman, 1996; Cooley, 1992). To facilitate change, Barnes and colleagues (Barnes & Walker, 1996) advise professionals and policy makers to start from the proposition that "authority deriving from professional knowledge is balanced by authority deriving from the experiential knowledge of the user. . . ." Empowerment does not remove the responsibilities of those who produce services, including responsibility to learn and change.

A recent example from the County of Devon in England shows the power of participation to change systems, to empower people to take more control over their care planning, and to save valuable professional resources for those who most need them (Searle, 2001). An outside study revealed that service users and caregivers found case management to be disempowering (something "done to them") and bureaucratic. The county's case management system was found to be not differentiated by need—i.e., both the more and less complex cases received case management. In response to the study, the county worked with service users, caregivers, and providers to create more partnering, enabling, and simple administrative procedures founded on the principles of more opportunity and access, building care plans on client strengths, providing good information and advice, and forming partnerships at all stages. The system that resulted started with a help desk to provide information and advice and some basic assessment and services in less complex cases. This was found to take care of 85% of all calls for help within 5 days without ever naming a case manager. After that, three levels of case management were available: self case management, care coordination, and extensive case management. Assignments were based on levels of need, risk, debility, and uncertainty. One empowering feature was to send the assessment document to users in advance. Caseloads dropped dramatically to 15 ongoing cases and five new cases. Other effects were more success at information and advice, shorter waiting lists, faster access to services, and more user and staff satisfaction.

Examples of Fully Integrated Systems

A real-world example of full integration in the United States is the Program for All-inclusive Care for the Elderly (PACE), which delivers, to a group of severally impaired elderly, all Medicare acute services and all Medicaid long-term care and ancillary services under capitated financing from both payers (Branch, Coulam, & Zimmerman, 1995; Eng et al., 1997; Irvin, Massey, & Dorsey, 1997; Kronick, Zhou, & Dreyfus, 1995; Rich, 1999). PACE focuses on a narrow group of highly vulnerable individuals who are poor enough to qualify for Medicaid, frail enough to meet nursing home eligibility criteria but still reside in the community, and willing to change doctors and receive all of their primary care services by regularly attending the PACE day health center. At the center, a team model of care delivers primary care, therapy, bathing, socialization, transportation, nutrition services, and more. In essence, PACE solves the financing part of the "square-round" dilemma by enrolling only those who are dually entitled, and it addresses other medical/community care differences by consolidating practice in the multi-disciplinary team.

In 1997 PACE was made a permanent option under Medicare, and the number of sites has grown steadily since then. In early 2001 there were 25 PACE programs (many with multiple day center sites) in 14 states serving 6,800 enrollees. An additional 10 programs in seven states serving 1,200 were in advanced stages of development (vanReenan, 2001). Most PACE sites are sponsored by hospitals, but a few are sponsored by HMOs. The federal evaluation found that PACE enrollees live longer, are more confident about life, attend more social activities, and have less hospital and nursing home use than a comparison group (Burstein, White, & Kidder, 1996).

The PACE model's major shortcoming is the narrowness of the frail, Medicaid-eligible population it serves; and numbers enrolled are further reduced by the requirement that enrolees change to the PACE physician and attend day care. Although Medicare beneficiaries not eligible for Medicaid are allowed to join, they must pay the several thousand dollars a month that Medicaid pays for long-term care. This has kept private enrollment very small. On a financial level, PACE programs are vulnerable to cuts in Medicare and Medicaid payment rates—particularly the latter, since a federal evaluation reported that Medicare realizes greater savings than Medicaid programs (Abt Associates, 1997).

A major initiative that is trying to build larger fully integrated systems is the Medicare/Medicaid Integration Program. Thirteen states have received grants and technical assistance to develop integrated systems for the full range of dual eligibles—from healthy to chronically ill, from community to nursing home residents. Besides the fact that targeting dual eligibles—as in PACE—solves the "square-round" challenge to integration, a key rationale for this targeting is the high need/cost profile of dual eligibles. In 1997 there were 6.7 million dual eligibles, representing 17% of the Medicare population but 28% of its spending and 19% of the Medicaid population but 35% of its spending (MMIP, 2001).

The path-breaking state for the Medicare/Medicaid initiative was Minnesota, which began voluntary enrollment in 1997 and three years later was serving 3,653 enrollees. This represented 25% of elderly dual eligibles in the Twin Cities and was in excess of enrollment targets (MMIP, 2001; Salisbury, 1997). However, the program's impact on community care services was more limited than this since 75% of the enrollees were nursing home residents, and many of these were conversions from the earlier EverCare Medicare nursing home demonstration.

The other states in the initiative have had difficulty duplicating Minnesota's achievements. Although compelling conceptually, dual eligible initiatives have been exceedingly difficult to implement because of long delays in working out Medicare and Medicaid regulatory conflicts, payment and risk arrangements, enrollment procedures, benefit packages, and more, all of which have led to long delays in obtaining Medicare and Medicaid waivers. Providers considering sponsoring a dual eligible program face complex planning and decision processes in deciding whether and how to participate in these initiatives (Ripley, 2001). The two other states with capitated/risk contracts for Medicaid services (Texas and Florida) were not able to arrange Medicare risk contracts with the same organizations. Several other states have received Medicare and Medicaid waivers but as of 2001 had not implemented or only partially implemented programs, partly because of shortages of willing providers (Massachusetts, Maine, New York, Colorado). Other states were still in the planning stage (Washington, New Hampshire, Rhode Island, Connecticut, Oregon) (MMIP, 2001). Another drawback is that many state models do not allow participating HMOs to enroll Medicare-only beneficiaries in a Social HMO option, which would expand the market substantially.

Examples of Coordinated Systems

An example of a model for coordinating medical and community care (with some integrated examples) is the Social HMO. It adds a finite package of expanded community care and short-term nursing facility benefits to an HMO via enhanced Medicare financing (Leutz et al., 1985). Social HMOs have much broader market potential than PACE, since like the Medicare/Medicaid dual eligible initiatives, they enroll both frail and non-frail elders. However, they are much broader than either since they include both dual eligible and Medicare-only members. As of 2002, four Social HMOs, including a site at Kaiser Permanente in the Northwest, were serving about 110,000 members, about 15% of whom had physical and cognitive disabilities that qualified them for the expanded community care benefits.

Three Social HMO sites that began in 1985 connect acute and community care services through case managers, who manage expanded community care benefits, maintain communication and referral points with acute care clinicians and care managers, and also facilitate access to other community care services. A second-round site that began in 1996 has moved toward full integration by forming interdisciplinary geriatric teams to coordinate care for the most complex members (Leutz, 2000). The importance of a coordinated approach is shown by the fact that referrals from the medical system contacts accounted for 50% to 70% of referrals to community care at Social HMO sites, with the rest divided about equally between self/family referrals and health screening (Altman et al., 1993).

Because the Social HMO fits relatively easily into an existing HMO, it is an appealing approach to better meet the needs of frail Medicare members. Social HMOs do not offer full coverage of long-term care benefits (as in PACE), but their coverage is still important. In 1999 the average spending across the four sites for all community care and service coordination was $51 per member per month, which compares favorably with spending in the rest of the public and private system (Table 1.3). Studies have shown that the limited community care benefit appears to provide adequate support for members unless they have extensive needs and weak family support (Leutz, Capitman, & Green, 2001). Also, Social HMOs may reduce permanent institutionalization by 40% or more (Boose, 1993; Fischer et al., 2001; Lutzky et al., 2000).

However, there are limitations to the Social HMO model. First, as in PACE, the Social HMO's financial success is tied both to the underlying level of Medicare payments to managed care plans, which were cut by the 1997 BBA (McBride, 1998), and to the adequacy of risk adjustors to protect plans against adverse selection on disability—the future of which is unresolved (MedPac, 1999). Low Medicare rates were one factor in the decision of one of the four original Social HMO sites to end operations in 1994 (Fischer et al., 1998; Leutz & Ripley, 1999). Second, while continuation of the Social HMO was endorsed in the 1997 BBA, Congress has not yet decided how to make Social HMOs a permanent option under Medicare+Choice. Finally, the Social HMO is available only for Medicare beneficiaries; it does not help other groups of people with disabilities.

Other Examples of Coordinated and Linked Systems

Less complicated than getting involved with Medicare and Medicaid waivers (as in PACE, Social HMOs, and dual eligible initiatives) is for health or community care systems to set up linkage and coordination on their own. A number of HMOs and hospital medical systems have tried to better connect their patients with community care services, generally in the context of trying to improve medical care for their most at-risk patients. Although most initiatives do not have all the characteristics of the general linkage and coordination models described above, they are illustrative of the challenges and opportunities in improving connections.

Even modest movements toward improved linkage can be important, since acute care providers are not formally required to make effective referrals to community care agencies providing long-term community care. This is in contrast to the built-in regulations under Medicare for acute care providers to refer to home health when it is needed and for skilled agency personnel to respond in a timely manner. Physicians' lack of knowledge and concern about functional status and community care is reflected in numerous studies:

- Physicians' assessments of the functional status of their patients were not in agreement with the patients' own assessments (Barker, Minneness, & Muller, 1998).
- 37% of patients over age 80 felt their clinician was unaware of their physical limitations; 42% of their emotional status; and 76% of their social needs. Half felt their care could be improved in these areas (Patterson et al., 1998).
- Primary care physicians made fewer diagnoses of Alzheimer's Disease than would seem indicated by their patient population, and they seldom referred to support services in the community (Brown et al., 1998).
- British primary care physicians were more knowledgeable about dementia diagnosing and managing dementia than expected, but they knew much less about community services: 30%–60% knew about day care, memory clinic, and support groups (Downs, 2001).
- Physician referrals to covered home health and nursing facilities were much more common than to community care services (adult day care, Alzheimer's Association, and aging network), although having a social worker or nurse in the office increased these referrals (Fortinsky, 1998). Caregiver issues were also often neglected.
- Typical geriatric assessments, health care information systems, and community services agencies collect data on caregivers' characteristics, such as their health status, their perceived need for assistance, and the status of their social support system (Anderson et al., 2000).
- Even in the Social HMO, frail patients often reported a "don't ask-don't tell" relationship with their physicians when it came to talking about their community care needs and services (Leutz, Capitman, & Green, 2001).

Several initiatives have tried to overcome physicians' limited concern with and connections to community care by adding linkage staff to physician practices. These precursors to KP's Manifesto 2005 demonstration provide important experience on approaches to identifying and engaging patients, as well as some indications of potential outcomes. For example, case management was featured in a 10-site demonstration of generalist physician's care for frail elders (Williams, n.d.). Three project examples show a case-manager-centered linkage model. First, a hospital-sponsored project linked physician offices to community care services through a social work coordinator in the office, who mailed a questionnaire to all over-65 visitors. Of 3,018 questionnaires, 815 were returned, and 62% of these needed follow up. Referrals were made to 2,256 community services for personal care and home health, durable medical equipment, transport, alternative housing, personal emergency response systems, and support groups. Seventy-five percent of the clients needed only two or three contacts by the liaison. A second project had control and experimental five-physician intern groups. An advanced practice nurse was assigned to the latter. Hospital admissions were reduced by 43% and ER use by 44%, with substantial net medical savings and improved patient satisfaction. A third project was a large non-profit medical group that added nurse case managers to primary care practices. Nurses supported physicians on complex cases and worked with patients and families, including linkage to community care services. The group experienced reductions in acute care, and the clinic decided to include the case management service in its risk plan.

In another study of a linkage model, a large California physicians group working with several Medicare HMOs added social work case managers randomly to 16 practices (3,480 older patients) but not to 19 control practices (2,929 patients). They identified case management patients through screening (58% to 63% return rates respectively), training of office staff to refer at-risk patients, and review of hospitalizations by a clinical nurse specialist. In the end only 3.2% of experimental patients received case management. There was slight, non-significant, net savings in acute costs (Boult et al., 2000).

In another example of linkage, a Connecticut HMO contracted with a care management group to do community care case management (including linkage to community care services) and also support primary care physicians in care of at risk elders. The contract included support from an advanced practice nurse for physicians with high numbers of elders. The HMO screened patients at admission and every two years. The case management agency also trained key acute system contacts to make referrals. A pilot study showed substantial medical savings after patients were referred to care management, but this may have been an artifact of the research design (Quinn, Prybylo, & Pannone, 1999).

Kaiser Permanente itself has been a leader in special care of high risk elders. This has included testing screening systems (Brody, Johnson, & Ried, 1997), special case management (IRCOA, 1990; Marshall et al., 1999), the Social HMO (Greenlick et al., 1988), and most recently the KP Care Management Institute's Eldercare Sourcebook. KP Mid-Atlantic provides an example of a linkage program for infants and children with disabilities. Early childhood educators were added to pediatric practices to provide parents of newborns with disabilities with information, support, and linkages to community services (Eggbeer, Littman, & Jones, 1997).

There are several common themes among these initiatives. First, they were built on models to support the work of the acute care system—e.g., to help physicians handle complex cases and to reduce system costs. Second, they included education and support to patients and families around the care plan. And third, the connections with community care services—although assumed—were not the central features of the project. In most projects, no data were reported on what community care services were received (data were generally not collected), and connecting with community care was seen as a professional rather than a systems activity. That is, the case manager apparently helped with linkage using his or her own knowledge of the community. With some exceptions, it did not seem to be an area in which investment seemed valued. The KP Manifesto 2005 demonstration went much farther in developing community care connections.

Looking at linkage initiated from the community care side, there are relatively few examples of community care service providers demonstrating linkage with medical care providers. Some large, multi-service long-term care providers—for example, members of the National Chronic Care Consortium—have linked by adding primary care capacity to their own systems. However, smaller community care agencies seldom have the power, the volume, or the funding to do the same. Nor is there state policy support. For example, a survey of 51 state aging programs found that only one required the formation of explicit formal links between health care providers (hospitals, physicians, and home health agencies) and the local agencies responsible for case management for aging network services (Leutz et al., 1992).

DISCUSSION

So what is an HMO to do if it wants to better serve the community care needs of its members with disabilities? Is this a problem that it should worry about at all, and, if so, for which members? Won't the family and public financing of community care services take care of things? How about the private insurance sector? Should an HMO sponsor PACE sites, wait for the Social HMO to be an option and offer that, and hope that its state initiates a dual eligible program? Or should it also or instead develop care coordination and linkage systems on its own both to better serve the medical care needs of all of its chronically ill and frail members, and to help them address community care needs? And how should the larger medical care system get involved, and what are the parallel changes needed in community care?

First, it is clear that need for support in community settings is widespread and differs by age, type of disability, and stage of life. It is also a major and sometimes stressful and unhealthy responsibility for family members (especially women). These needs are only going to grow. Medical care providers are put on the spot when their patients have community care needs, if only because the conditions that foster medical care system encounters also often foster disability. Medical care providers and insurers can (and do) protect their spaces against incursions of long-term care needs, but that does not make the needs go away.

Second, there are few if any states or localities in the United States where community care services are easily accessed by all who need them. Skilled home health care covered by health insurance is important, but many patients still need help with ADLs and IADLs when skilled care expires, and even more never qualify for skilled care in the first place. And the biggest single skilled care payer—Medicare—has recently cut way back on long-term cases. Public and private financing of non-skilled community care services is fragmented, rife with no-care zones, haves and have-nots, long waiting lists, high costs for those who fail to qualify, and high family responsibilities for anyone with a caring family but no private funds. For some populations, some states and localities have single-entry access points to coordinate applications to and delivery of those publicly funded services that are available, but separation of programming by funding source is more likely the rule.

Third, despite the fragmentation and gaps in the community care system, some types of help are available in virtually all communities, through public, private, self-help, and volunteer sources. For many people, especially those with strong family support, just a little formal help or short-term intensive help can make a difference.

Fourth, left to their own devices and interests, most medical care providers do not know a lot about community care services and do not do much to connect their patients to them. This is not a condemnation, especially of busy physicians with unique skills. It's just a fact that dealing with functional status deficits is not seen as a primary clinical issue, and that perspective has been difficult to change in most acute/long-term care integration efforts. Feeling like "your integration is my fragmentation" is an understandable reaction for a busy physician who has unique and important responsibilities.

Fifth, the major U.S. payers for people who are old and disabled—Medicare and Medicaid—do not have a ready answer for better connecting medical care and community care. Demonstrations of full Medicare/Medicaid integration have been very difficult to pull off, and most of those that are operating are serving small and narrow populations. High need and utilization profiles make these important populations to serve with integrated programming, but they fulfill just a piece of an HMO's mission to serve all of its members with disabilities. The Social HMO reaches a larger potential market, but its future is uncertain. And even if the Social HMO is added as a Medicare program option, it is limited to Medicare beneficiaries, and its feasibility depends on continued idiosyncratic Medicare reimbursement and regulatory arrangements in general, and on local Medicare supplement market conditions in particular.

Sixth, linkage and coordination generated from the medical care side has the potential to reach virtually any chosen population that is at risk of chronic illness and disability. Although public and philanthropic priorities for targeting have shaped many such initiatives to date, theoretically a medical care system could try to target all important types of chronic illness and disability with special internal supports such as case management plus external community care to families and for connections to community services. This could be the basis for a community-oriented, public health system of care that has been advocated as an alternative to divided and institution-oriented approaches (Andersen & Pourat, 1997). A decision to pursue a type of linked/coordinated system was recently made in Israel, which is pursuing a commission recommendation to create a single point of contact for the public in the same building (geographic proximity). It will force inter-professional cooperation through a single assessment and other integrating components (Brodsky, 2001). England also is pursuing national directives to better coordinate community care and medical care under the government's "modernization" initiative.

Seventh, the weaknesses of the medically-based linkage/coordination model are important. Someone needs to pay for screening, case management, support to primary care, and so forth. "Integration costs before it pays," and managers under budgetary constraints are not likely to front the money on the promise of future savings. Also, unlike the integration models that pool Medicare and Medicaid and/or private funds to finance new community care benefits, little or no new funding for community care services is created. Therefore, linkage case managers and referral staff need to rely on existing community services. The review of the numerous gaps in the financing and delivery of community care services brings to mind a common piece of gallows humor among community care service veterans: "All assessed and nowhere to go." Is this the end game for the linkage model?

This final concern turned out to be one of the keys to success or failure for KP's Manifesto 2005 demonstration. The vision of including community care services for all of its members with disabilities by 2005 almost totally relied on the existence of community care services in the community and on members' being able to access those services through their own funds, public funds, or other private sources. Because the community connections were so important to success, demonstration designers decided to target funds toward building those connections rather than toward internal case management, which KP had already developed in earlier initiatives.

The demonstration's linkage activities turned out to go beyond learning about local community care resources and making good referrals. They brought KP into joint efforts with a wide range of community care agencies to think through and try out new ways of working together much more closely around service to shared clients. This is a model that builds on the prior reform efforts reviewed in this chapter, but it goes beyond what any U.S. health care system and community agencies have done before. In the process, KP and the agencies learned a great deal about themselves, each other, the individuals they jointly served, and how complex it can be to create linked and coordinated systems. The chapters that follow show that their efforts were not always successful, but both successes and failures hold valuable lessons for the future.

Voltaire had the insight that "The best is the enemy of the good." ("Le mieux est l'ennemi du bien.") Looking over the 30-year search for why and how to expand funding for community care services for persons with disabilities, one wonders if this wisdom applies. Has the search for the ideal community care program kept us from recognizing and more widely adopting good ones? Have efforts to fully integrate financing and services for the most in-need and most expensive diverted attention from doing something more modest for a much, much larger number of people with less intensive needs and less expensive service profiles? The efforts of the KP demonstration sites and the agencies and members they worked with did not reach the ideal, but they did begin to show what a "good" health care system for people with disabilities can look like.

REFERENCES

American Association for Retired Persons (ARRP). (1995). *Home and community-based long-term care.* Washington, DC: Center on Elderly People Living Alone.

Abrahams, R., Capitman, J. A., Leutz, W., & Macko, P. (1989). Variations in care planning in the Social/HMO: A qualitative study. *Gerontologist, 29*(16), 725–736.

Abt Associates. (1997). *A comparison of the PACE capitation rates to projected costs in the first year of enrollment.* Evaluation Report. Cambridge, MA: Abt.

Alecxih, L. M. B., Corea, J., & Kennell, D. L. (1995). Implications of health care financing, delivery, and benefit design for persons with disabilities. In J. M. Wiener, S. B. Clauser, & D. L. Kennell (Eds.), *Persons with disabilities: Issues in health care financing and service delivery.* Washington, DC: The Brookings Institution.

Altman, S., Leutz, W., Capitman, J., Abrahams, R., Hallfors, D., Ritter, G., & Gruenberg, L. (1993). *Design of Second-Generation Social HMO Sites.* Waltham, MA: Brandeis University Institute for Health Policy. Report to Health Care Financing Administration.

Andersen, R., & Pourat, N. (1997). Toward a synthesis of a public health agenda for an aging society. In T. Hickey, M. Speers, & T. Prohaska (Eds.), *Public health and aging.* Baltimore: The Johns Hopkins University Press.

Anderson, R., Bradham, D., Jackson, S., Heuser, M., Wofford, J., & Colombo, K. (2000). Caregivers' unmet needs for support in caring for functionally impaired elderly persons: A community sample. *Journal of Health Care for the Poor and Underserved, 11*(4), 412–429.

Anthony, C. R., Zarit, S. H., & Gatz, M. (1998). Symptoms of psychological distress among caregiver of dementia patients. *Psychology and Aging, 3,* 245–248.

Archbold, P. G., & Stewart, B. J. (1988). *The effects of organized caregiver relief.* (Report to NCNR, R01 NU/AG 01140). Portland, OR: Oregon Health Sciences University.

Archbold, P. G., & Stewart, B. J. (1996). The nature of the caregiving role and nursing interventions for caregiving families. In E. A. Swanson & T. Tripp-Reimer (Eds.), *Advances in Gerontological Nursing* (pp. 133–156). New York: Springer.

Archbold, P. G., Stewart, B. J., et al. (1990). Mutuality and preparedness as predictors of caregiver role strain. *Research in Nursing and Health, 13,* 375–384.

Archbold, P. G., Stewart, B. J., Greenlick, M. R., & Harvath, T. A. (1992). The clinical assessment of mutuality and preparedness in family caregivers to frail older people. In S. G. Funk, E. M. Tornquist, M. T. Champagne, & L. A. Copp (Eds.), *Key aspects of elder care.* New York: Springer.

Baldwin, S., & Twigg, J. (1991). Women and community care—reflections on a debate. In M. Maclean & D. Groves (Eds.), *Women's issues in social policy.* London: Routledge.

Barker, J. C., Minneness, L. S., & Muller, H. B. (1998). Older home health care patients and their physicians: Assessment of functional ability. *Home Health Care Services Quarterly, 17*(2), 21–39.

Barnes, M., & Prior, D. (1996). Spoilt for choice? How consumerism can disempower public service users. *Public Money and Management, 15*(3), 53–58.

Barnes, M., & Walker, A. (1996). Consumerism versus empowerment: A principled approach to the involvement of older service users. *Policy and Politics, 24*(2), 375–393.

Barton, L. (1993). The struggle for citizenship: The case of disabled people. *Disability and Society, 8*(3), 235–248.

Batavia, A. I. (1993). Health care reform and people with disabilities. *Health Affairs* (Spring), 40–56.

Batavia, A, I., DeJong, G., & McKnew, L. B. (1991). Toward a national personal assistance program: The independent living model of long-term care for persons with disabilities. *Journal of Health Politics, Policy and Law, 16*(3), 523–545.

Bewley, C., & Glendinning, C. (1994). Representing the views of disabled people in care planning. *Disability and Society, 9*(3), 301–314.

Bishop, C., Kerwin, J., & Wallack, S. (1999). The Medicare home health benefit: Implications of recent payment changes. *Care Management Journals, 1*(3), 189–196.

Bishop, C., & Skwara, K. C. (1993). Recent growth in Medicare home health. *Health Affairs* (Fall), 95–110.

Blackman, D. K., Brown, T. E., & Leaner, R. N. (1986). Four years of a community long term care project: The South Carolina experience. *Pride Institute Journal, 3,* 30–49.

Boose, L. (1993). A study of the differences between social HMO and other Medicare beneficiaries enrolled in Kaiser Permanente under capitation contracts regarding intermediate care facility user rates and expenditures. Portland Oregon: Portland State University.

Boult, C., Rassen, J., Rassen, A., Moore, R., & Robison, S. (2000). The effect of case management on the costs of health care for enrollees in Medicare Plus Choice plans: A randomized trial. *Journal of the American Geriatrics Society, 48*(8), 996–1001.

Branch, L., Coulam, R., & Zimmerman, Y. (1995). The PACE evaluation: Initial findings. *Gerontologist, 35*(3), 349–359.

Brodsky, J. (2001). Improving the system of care for the elderly in a changing health care environment. Paper read at 17th Congress of the International Gerontology Association, July 3, 2001, at Vancouver, Canada.

Brody, K., Johnson, R. E., & Ried, D. L. (1997). Evaluation of a self-report screening instrument to predict frailty outcomes in aging populations. *The Gerontologist, 37*(2), 182–191.

Brown, C. J., Mutran, E. J., Sloane, P. D., & Long, K. M. (1998). Primary care physicians' knowledge and behavior related to Alzheimer's Disease. *Journal of Applied Gerontology, 17*(4), 462–479.

Burstein, N. R., White, A. J., & Kidder, D. (1996). Evaluation of the PACE Demonstration: The impact of PACE on participant outcomes. Cambridge, MA: Abt Associates.

Callahan, J. J. (2000). Do we need a Surgeon General's report on home and community based services? *Gerontologist,* 5–6.

Capitman, J., Abrahams, R., & MacAdam, M. (1990). Case management in emerging long-term care systems. In P. Katz, R. Kane, & M. Mezey (Eds.), *Advances in long-term care.* New York: Springer Publishing.

Capitman, J., & Sciegaj, M. (1995). A contextual approach for understanding individual autonomy in managed community long-term care. *Gerontologist, 35*(4), 533–540.

Cassel, C. K., Rudberg, M. A., & Olshansky, S. J. (1992). The price of success: Health care in an aging society. *Health Affairs,* Summer, 86–99.

Clark, F., Azen, S., Zemke, R., et al. (1997). Occupational therapy for independent-living older adults. *Journal of the American Medical Association, 278*(16), 1321–1326.

Clark, H., Dyer, S., & Hartman, L. (1996). *Going home: Older people leaving the hospital.* London: Joseph Rowntree Foundation.

Coleman, E. A., Kramer, A. M., Kowalsky, J. C., Eckhoff, D., Lin, M., Hester, E. J., Morgenstern, N., & Steiner, J. F. (2000). A comparison of functional outcomes after hop fracture in group/staff HMOs and fee-for-service systems. *Effective Clinical Practice, 3*(5), 229–239.

Committee on Ways and Means. (1996). *The Green Book.* U.S. House of Representatives.

Cooley, W. C. (1992). Natural beginnings—unnatural encounters: Events a the outset for families of children with disabilities. In J. Nisbet (Ed.), *Natural supports in school, at work and in the community for people with severe disabilities.* Baltimore: Paul H. Brookes Publishing Co.

Coppel, D. B., Burton, C., Becker, J., & Fiore, J. (1985). Relationships of cognition and associated coping reactions to depression in spousal caregiver of Alzheimers Disease. *Cognitive Therapy and Research, 9,* 253–266.

Crown, W., Burwell, B., & Alecxih, L. (1994). An analysis of asset testing for nursing home benefits. Washington, DC: AARP Public Policy Institute.

Crown, W., Capitman, J., & Leutz, W. (1992). Economic rationality, the market for private long-term care insurance, & the role for public policy. *The Gerontologist, 32*(4), 478–485.

Davis, M., & O'Brien, E. (1996). Profile of persons with disabilities in Medicare and Medicaid. *Health Care Financing Review, 17*(4), 179–212.

Deimling, G. T., & Bass, D. M. (1986). Symptoms of mental impairment among elderly adults and their effects on their caregivers. *Journal of Gerontology, 41, 778–784.*

Doty, P. (2000). *Cost-effectiveness of home and community-based long-term care services.* Washington DC: U.S. Dept of Health and Human Services. Asst. Secretary for Planning and Evaluation.

Doty, P., Jackson, M. E., & Crown, W. (1998). The impact of female caregivers' employment status on patterns of formal and informal eldercare. *The Gerontologist, 38*(3), 331–341.

Doty, P., Matthias, R., & Franke, T. (1999). In-home supportive services for the elderly and disabled: A comparison of client-directed and professional management models of service delivery. Washington DC: U.S. Dept of Health and Human Services.

Downs, M. (2001). An intervention to improve primary care practitioners' response to people with dementia and their families. Paper read at 17th Congress of the International Gerontology Association, July 3, 2001, at Vancouver, Canada.

Eggbeer, L., Littman, C. L., & Jones, M. (1997). Zero to Three's developmental specialist in pediatric practice project: An important support for parents and young children. *Zero to Three,* (June/July), 3–8.

Eggert, G. M., Zimmer, J. G., Hall, W. J., & Friedman, B. (1991). Case management: A randomized controlled study comparing a neighborhood team and a centralized individual model. *Health Services Research, 26*(4), 471–507.

Emanuel, E. J., Fairclough, D. L., Slutsman, J., & Emanuel, L. L. (2000). Understanding economic and other burdens of terminal illness: The experience of patients and their caregivers. *Annals of Internal Medicine, 132*(6), 451–459.

Eng, C., Pedulla, J., Eleazer, P. G., McCann, R., & Fox, N. (1997). Program of All-inclusive Care for the Elderly (PACE): An innovative model of integrated geriatric care and financing. *Journal of the American Geriatrics Society, 45*(2), 223–232.

England, S., Kiegher, S., Miller, B., & Linsk, N. (1991). Community care policies and gender justice. In M. Minkler & C. Estes (Eds.), *Critical perspectives on aging: The political and moral economy of growing old.* Amityville, NY: Baywood Publishing Company.

Evers, A. (1994). Payments for care: A small but significant part of a wider debate. In A. Evers, M. Pijl, & C. Ungerson (Eds.), *Payments for care.* Brookfield, VT: Ashgate Publishing Co.

Evers, A. (1995). The future of elderly care in Europe: Limits and aspirations. In T. Scharf & C. C. Wenger (Eds.), *International perspectives on community care for older people.* Brookfield, VT: Ashgate.

Farkas, J. I., & Himes, C. L. (1997). The influence of caregiving and employment on the voluntary activities of midlife and older women. *Journal of Gerontology: Social Sciences, 52B*(4), S180–189.

Fischer, L. R., & Eustis, N. (1994). Family caregivers and home care workers. In E. Kahana, D. E. Biegel, & M. L. Wykle (Eds.), *Family caregiving across the lifespan.* Thousand Oaks, CA: Sage Publications.

Fischer, L. R., Green, C. A., Goodman, M., Aickin, M., Brody, K. K., Wei, F., Phelps, L. W., & Leutz, W. N. (2001). Community-based care and risk of nursing home placement. Paper read at American Association of Health Plans Research Conference, April 2001, at Seattle, WA.

Fischer, L. R., Wisner, C., Leutz, W., Miller, A., von Sternberg, T., & Ripley, J. (1998). The closing of a Social HMO: A case study. *Journal of Aging and Social Policy, 10*(1), 57–76.

Fortinsky, R. H. (1998). How linked are physicians to community support services for their patients with dementia? *Journal of Applied Gerontology, 17*(4), 480–498.

GAO. (1993). Long-term care insurance: High percentage of policy holders drop policies. U.S. General Accounting Office.

Gerry, M. H., & Mirsky, A. J. (1992). Guiding principles for public policy on natural supports. In J. Nisbet (Ed.), *Natural supports in school, at work and in the community for people with severe disabilities.* Baltimore: Paul H. Brookes Publishing Co.

Glendinning, C., & Lloyd, B. (1997). *Developing local "continuing care" policies and guidelines: The implications for primary and community health services.* National Primary Care Research and Development Center—University of Manchester.

Goodwin, J. S. (1999). Geriatrics and the limits of modern medicine. *New England Journal of Medicine, 340*(16), 1283–1285.

Greene, V., Ondrich, J., & Laditka, S. (1998). Can home care services achieve cost savings in long-term care for older people? *Journal of Gerontology: Social Sciences, 53B*(4), S228–S238.

Greenlick, M. R., & Brody, K. K. (1997). Home health services in a managed-care system. In D. M. Fox & C. Raphael (Eds.), *Home-based care for a new century.* Copublished by Blackwell and Milbank Memorial Fund.

Greenlick, M. R., Nonnenkamp, L., Gruenberg, L., Leutz, W., & Lamb, S. (1988). The S/HMO demonstration: Policy implications for long term care in HMOs. *Pride Institute Journal, 7*(3), 15–24.

Guralnik, J. M., LaCroix, A. Z., Everett, D. F., & Kovar, M. G. (1989). *Aging in the eighties: The prevalence of comorbidity and its association with disability.* Malden, MA: National Center for Health Statistics.

Hallfors, D., Leutz, W., Capitman, J., & Ritter, G. (1994). Stability of frailty in the social/health maintenance organization. *Health Care Financing Review, 15*(3), 1–12.

Harrington, M. (1998). The care equation. *The American Prospect,* (39), 61–67.

Holstein, M., & Cole, T. (1996). The evolution of long-term care in America. In R. Binstock, L. Cluff, & O. V. Mering (Eds.), *The future of long-term care.* Baltimore, MD: Johns Hopkins University Press.

IRCOA. (1990). Guide to the Model of Care for Older Members. Portland, OR: Interregional Committee on Aging, Model of Care Subcommittee, Kaiser Permanente.

Irvin, C. V., Massey, S., & Dorsey, T. (1997). Determinants of enrollment among applicants to PACE. *Health Care Financing Review, 19*(2), 135–153.

Kassner, E., & Martin, J. (1996). Decisions, decisions: Service allocation in home and community-based long-term care programs—a four-state analysis. AARP Public Policy Institute.

Kemper, P., Applebaum, R. A., & Harrigan, M. (1987). Community care demonstrations: What have we learned? *Health Care Financing Review, 8*(4), 87–100.

Kiecolt-Glaser, J. K., & Glaser, R. (1999). Chronic stress and mortality among older adults. *Journal of the American Medical Association, 282*(23), 225–226.

Knight, B. G., Lutzky, S. M., & Macofsky-Urban, F. (1993). A meta analytic review of interventions for caregiver distress: Recommendations for future research. *The Gerontologist, 33,* 240–248.

Komisar, H. L., & Feder, J. (1998). The Balanced Budget Act of 1997: Effects on Medicare's home health benefit and beneficiaries who need long-term care. Washington DC: Georgetown University Institute for Health Care Research and Policy.

Krauss, L. E., Stoddard, S., & Gilmartin, D. (1996). Chartbook on disability in the United States. National Institute on Disability and Rehabilitation Research.

Kronick, R., Zhou, Z., & Dreyfus, A. (1995). Making risk adjustment work for everyone. *Inquiry,* (Spring).

Laudicina, S. S., & Burwell, B. (1988). A profile of Medicaid home and community-based care waivers, 1985: Findings of a national survey. *Journal of Health, Politics, & Law, 13,* 525–546.

LaPlante, M. P., & Carlson, D. (1996). Disability in the US: Prevalence and causes, 1992. San Francisco CA: University of CA, Institute of Health and Aging, Disability Statistics Rehabilitation Research and Training Center.

Leutz, W. (1998). Home care benefits for persons with disabilities. *American Rehabilitation, 24*(3), 6–14.

Leutz, W. (1999). Five laws for integrating medical and social care: Lessons from the US and UK. *The Milbank Memorial Fund Quarterly, 77*(1), 77–110.

Leutz, W. (2000). Social HMO Progress Report. Waltham, MA: Social HMO Consortium, Brandeis University.

Leutz, W., Capitman, J., & Green, C. (2001). A limited entitlement for community care: How members use services. *Journal of Aging and Social Policy, 12*(3), 43–64.

Leutz, W. N., Capitman, J. C., MacAdam, M., & Abrahams, R. (1992). *Care for frail elders: Developing community solutions.* New York: Auburn House.

Leutz, W., & Ripley, J. (1999). Reply to commentary on the closing of a social HMO. *Journal of Aging and Social Policy,* Forthcoming.

Leutz, W., Sciegaj, M., & Capitman, J. (1997). Client-centered case management: A survey of state programs. *Journal of Case Management, 6*(1), 18–25.

Leutz, W. N., Greenberg, J. N., Abrahams, R., Prottas, J., Diamond, L. M., & Gruenberg, L. (1985). *Changing health care for an aging society: Planning for the social health maintenance organization.* Lexington, MA: Lexington Books.

Levine, C. (1999). The loneliness of the long-term care giver. *New England Journal of Medicine, 340*(20), 1587–1590.

Litvak, S., & Kennedy, J. (1991). Case studies of six state personal assistance service programs funded by the Medicaid personal care option. World Institute on Disability.

Litwak, E., Jessop, D. J., & Moulton, H. J. (1994). Optimal use of formal and informal systems over the life course. In E. Kahana, D. E. Biegel, & M. L. Wykle (Eds.), *Family caregiving across the lifespan.* Thousand Oaks, CA: Sage Publications.

Liu, K., Hanson, J., & Coughlin, T. (1995). Characteristics and outcomes of persons screened into Connecticut's 2176 program. In J. M. Wiener, S. B. Clauser, & D. L. Kennell (Eds.), *Persons with disabilities: Issues in health care financing and service delivery.* Washington, DC: The Brookings Institution.

Liu, K., Wissoker, D., & Rimes, C. (1998). Determinants and costs of Medicare postacute care provided by SNFs and HHAs. *Inquiry, 35*(1), 49–61.

Long, S. K. (1995). Combining formal and informal care in serving frail elderly persons. In J. M. Wiener, S. B. Clauser, & D. L. Kennell (Eds.), *Persons with disabilities: Issues in health care financing and service delivery.* Washington, DC: The Brookings Institution.

Lutzky, S., Browning, N., Alecxih, L. M. B., Neill, C., & Mignone, B. (2000). *Assessing the impact of the SCAN Social HMO on long nursing facility stays.* Falls Church, VA: The Lewin Group.

Marshall, B., Long, M., Voss, J., Demma, K., & Skerl, K. P. (1999). Case management of the elderly in a HMO: The implications for program administration under managed care. *Journal of Healthcare Management, 44*(6), 477–491.

Mauser, E. (1997). Medicare home health initiatives: Current activities and future directions. *Health Care Financing Review, 18*(3), 275–291.

McBride, T. D. (1998). Disparities in access to Medicare managed care plans and their benefits. *Health Affairs, 17*(6), 170–180.

McCall, N., Bauer, E. J., & Korb, J. (1996). *Participation of private insurers in the partnerships for long-term care.* San Francisco: Laguna Research Associates.

Medpac. (1999). Report to Congress: Selected Medicare Issues (Chapter 5: Managed care for frail Medicare beneficiaries). Washington, DC: Medicare Payment Advisory Committee.

Mitchell, E. (1996). *A legislator's guide to Medicaid waivers.* Portland, ME: National Academy for State Health Policy.

MMIP (2001). Minnesota Senior Health Options Program Overview. College Park, MD: Center on Aging. Medicare/Medicaid Integration Program

Morgan, R. O., Virnig, B. A., DeVito, C. A., & Persily, N. A. (1997). The Medicare HMO revolving door—the healthy go in and the sick go out. *New England Journal of Medicine, 337*(3), 169–175.

Naylor, M. D., Brooten, D., Campbell, R., Jacobsen, B. S., Mezey, M. D., Pauly, M. N., & Schwartz, J. S. (1999). Comprehensive discharge planning and home follow-up of hospitalized elders. *Journal of the American Medical Association, 281*(7), 613–620.

NCOA (1997). Cash and counseling: Who will choose it? In *Consumer Choice News,* National Council on Aging.

Newcomer, R., Yordi, C., DuNah, R., Fox, P., & Wilkinson, A. (1999). Effects of the Medicare Alzheimer's Disease demonstration on caregiver burden and depression. *Health Services Research, 34*(3), 669–690.

OIG (1999). Medicare beneficiary access to home health agencies. Washington, DC: Office of the Inspector General, Department of Health and Human Services.

Patterson, J. A., Bierman, A., & Splaine, M. (1998). The population of people age 80 and over: A sentinel group for understanding the future of health care in the U.S. *Journal of Ambulatory Care Management, 21*(3), 10–16.

Pavalko, E. K., & Artis, J. E. (1997). Women's caregiving and paid work: Causal relationships in late midlife. *Journal of Gerontology: Social Sciences, 52B*(4), S1170–179.

Pepper Commission. (1990). A call for action. U.S. Bipartisan Commission on Comprehensive Health Care.

Quinn, J. L., Prybylo, M., & Pannone, P. (1999). Community care management across the continuum. *Care Management Journals, 1*(4), 223–231.

Rabiner, D. J., Arcury, T. A., Howard, H. A., & Copeland, K. A. (1997). The perceived availability, quality, & cost of long-term care services in America. *Journal of Aging and Social Policy, 9*(3), 43–65.

Retchin, S. M., Clement, D. G., Rossiter, L. F., Brown, S., Brown, R., & Nelson, L. (1992). How the elderly fare in HMOs: Outcomes from the Medicare competition demonstrations. *Health Services Research, 27*(5), 651–669.

Rich, M. L. (1999). The PACE model: Description and impressions of a capitated model of long-term care for the elderly. *The Care Management Journals, 1*(1), 62–70.

Ripley, J. (2001, June). Coordinating care for the dual-eligible population. *Healthcare Financial Management*, 39–43.

Rivlin, A. M., & Wiener, J. (1988). *Caring for the disabled elderly: Who will pay?* The Brookings Institution.

Rodat, C., Griesbach, F., & Zadoorian, J. (1997). New York State home care: A system at risk. *The Journal of Long Term Home Health Care, 16*(4), 2–16.

Rosenbaum, S. (2000). The Olmstead decision: Implications for state health policy. *Health Affairs, 19*(5), 228–232.

Ruchlin, H. S., Morris, J. N., & Eggert, G. M. (1982). Sounding Boards. Management and financing of long-term-care services: A new approach to a chronic problem. *New England Journal of Medicine, 306*(2), 101–106.

Salisbury, J. (1997). Acute, long-term care providers team up to manage Minnesota's dual eligibles. *State Health Watch, 4*(12), 3–6.

Schlenker, R., Shaughnessy, P., & Hittle, D. (1995, Fall). Patient-level cost of home health care under capitated and fee-for-service payment. *Inquiry, 32*, 252–270.

Schnelle, J. F. (1999). Objective and subjective measures of the quality of managed care in nursing homes. *Medical Care, 37*(4), 375–383.

Schorr, A. (1992). *The personal social services: An outside view.* Joseph Rowntree Foundation.

Schulz, R., & Beach, S. R. (1999). Caregiving as a risk factor for mortality. *Journal of the American Medical Association, 282*(23), 2215–2219.

Searle, P. (2001). Modernizing care management in the United Kingdom. Paper read at Fifth International Care/Case Management Conference, July 1, 2001, at Vancouver, Canada.

Shaughnessy, P., Schlenker, R., & Hittle, D. (1994). Home health care outcomes under capitated and fee-for-service payment. *Health Care Financing Review, 16*(1), 187–222.

Shaughnessy, P., Schlenker, R. E., Crisler, K. S., Arnold, A. G., Powell, M. C., &

Beaudry, J. M. (1996). Home care: Moving forward with continuous quality improvement. *The Journal of Aging and Social Policy, 7*(3/4), 149–168.

Simon-Rusinowitz, L., Mahoney, K. J., Desmond, S. M., Shjopop, D. M., Squillace, M. R., & Fay, R. A. (1997). Determining consumer preferences for a cash option: Arkansas survey results. *Health Care Financing Review, 19*(2), 73–96.

Small, G. W., Rabns, P. V., Barry, P. P., Buckholz, N. S., DeKosky, S. T., et al. (1997). Diagnosis and treatment of Alzheimer Disease and related disorders. *Journal of the American Medical Society, 278*(16), 1363–1371.

Smith, D. M., Weinberger, M., Katz, B. P., & Moore, P. S. (1988, July). Postdischarge care and readmissions. *Medical Care, 26,* 699–708.

Smith, J. E., & Smith, D. L. (2000). No map. No guide. *Care Management Journals, 2*(1), 27–33.

Stone, D. (2000). *Reframing home health care policy.* Cambridge, MA: Radcliffe Public Policy Center.

Tennstedt, S. L., Crawford, S. L., & McKinlay, J. B. (1993). Is family care on the decline? A longitudinal investigation of the substitution of formal long-term care services for informal care. *Milbank Quarterly, 71*(4), 601–624.

Thomas, C. P., & Payne, S. M. C. (1998). Home alone: Unmet need for formal support services among home health clients. *Home Health Services Quarterly, 17*(2), 1–20.

Twigg, J., & Atkin, K. (1994). *Carers perceived, policy and practice in informal care.* Buckingham: Open University Press.

vanReenan, C. (2001). Personal communication.

Walker, A. (1984). Community care and the elderly in Great Britain: Theory and practice. In M. Minkler & C. Estes (Eds.), *Readings in the political economy of aging.* Amityville, NY: Baywood Publishing Co.

Ware, J. E., Bayliss, M. S., Rogers, W. H., Kosinski, M., & Tarlov, A. R. (1996). Differences in 4-year health outcomes for elderly and poor, chronically ill patients treated in HMO and fee-for-service systems. *Journal of the American Medical Association, 276*(13), 1039–1047.

Weissert, W. G., & Cready, C. M. (1989). Toward a model for improved targeting of aged at risk of institutionalization. *Health Services Research, 24*(4), 485–310.

Weissert, W. G., Cready, C. M., & Pawelak, J. E. (1988). The past and future of home and community-based long-term Care. *Milbank Quarterly, 66*(2), 309–388.

Welch, H. G., Wennberg, D. E., & Welch, W. P. (1996). The use of Medicare home health care services. *The New England Journal of Medicine, 335*(5), 324–329.

Wiener, J., & Skaggs, J. (1995). Current approaches to integrating acute and LTC financing and services. AARP Public Policy Institute.

Wiener, J., & Sullivan, C. M. (1995). Long-term care for the younger population: A policy synthesis. In J. M. Wiener, S. B. Clauser, & D. L. Kennell (Eds.), *Persons with disabilities: Issues in health care financing and service delivery.* Washington, DC: The Brookings Institution.

Williams, B. C., & Weissert, W. G. (1994). ADL dependent people may also be sick: Neglect of the "home health" population in the home care debate. *Home Health Services Quarterly, 14*(4), 23–35.

Williams, F. N. D. The John A. Hartford Generalist Physician Initiative Report. Tempe, AZ: Arizona State University School of Health Administration and Policy.

Yelin, E. H., Criuswell, L. A., & Feigenbaum, P. G. (1996). Health care utilization and outcomes among persons with rheumatoid arthritis in fee-for-service and group practice settings. *Journal of the American Medical Association, 276*(13), 1048–1053.

Yordi, C. L. (1991). Case management practice in the SHMO demonstrations. Berkeley Planning Associates and the University of California San Francisco.

2

Manifesto 2005

Walter Leutz, Merwyn Greenlick, and Kathy Brody

> By the year 2005 Kaiser Permanente will have expanded its scope of services to include a broad range of home- and community-based services that would be easily accessible to persons with functional disabilities. This will be a multi-disciplinary system with providers and consumers of care working in collaboration to maximize the independent function of persons with disabilities of any age.

Manifesto 2005 stakes out a bold vision for an HMO, whose primary business after all is the delivery of acute medical care. Expanding services, including community care, and addressing issues related to disability are not the directions in which most health care providers and insurers are heading. But the history of Kaiser Permanente (KP) shows that the Manifesto was just the next step in an earlier series of planned, system-wide initiatives to understand the needs growing numbers of elders and other members with chronic illnesses, and to take steps to improve their care. These initiatives created and tested new approaches, particularly in the area of coordinated care for frail members residing in their homes and other community settings. Thus the Manifesto, and the decision of KP leadership to invest in a demonstration to test its vision, were consistent KP's history of innovation.

As Chapter 1 shows, the dilemma that KP faced in choosing ways to strengthen care for members with disabilities was that the current models for expanding the scope and coordination of services were either flawed, narrow, or self-limiting. On one side, the health-system based approaches tended not to recognize the medical model's inability to address personal and social care needs. On the other, models that expanded community care generally focused on a narrow segment of the population defined by income, age or functional status. Moreover, states varied in their interest in such services, which meant that what the health plan could do, would vary widely by region. Finally, financing was a problem: There was not a model available for the health plan to bring community care services to the full range of members with disabilities without significant new financing.

Thus, the Manifesto was audacious: declare that these are services your members need; commit to consider them as part of clinical practice; and do something to make them available. At a time when HMOs were being accused of avoiding the oldest and sickest Medicare beneficiaries, and when fears were being expressed about how well the disabled would fare in HMOs (Batavia, 1993), how and why did the nation's largest and oldest HMO decide to step forward? What had been the health plan's experience with services for frail and disabled members that informed the development of the Manifesto? The first section of this chapter provides this KP history and background.

Once the Manifesto was adopted, the community care demonstration was conceived, organized, and implemented quickly. Internal health plan funding and the use of the existing interregional committee structure helped speed the process. Yet it was not clear at the outset exactly what would be demonstrated. The Manifesto listed community care services and set the goal of access, but there was no model articulated for making this happen. Who would pay for these new services? How could community care be made available if it couldn't be paid for by the health plan? Who would deliver the service? Which members would be eligible, and who would decide what services they needed? The second section of the chapter describes the development of the demonstration, from the drafting of the Manifesto to the RFP (request for proposal) and site selection.

It was during the course of reviewing applications and setting final review criteria that practical approaches emerged for accessing community care. The model that eventually evolved was based on a few simple propositions that were consistent with linkage and care coordination levels of integration described in Chapter 1: (a) rely on existing community care systems and financing, (b) focus health plan efforts on making better connections with those systems and services for members, and (c) develop a new service internally only if it is not readily available in the community.

The 15 projects that were funded (composed of 32 sites, since some projects were multi-site) cut overlapping paths across the fields of community care and its clients. The third section of the chapter provides an overview of the projects by summarizing their goals, target members, locations, and funding from the demonstration. This serves as an introduction to the next four chapters, in which projects are detailed as examples of how to link with community care agencies, how to connect with members, how to make internal changes at in the health plan, and how to devise linkage projects for members younger than 65.

The final piece of the puzzle was evaluation. Kaiser Permanente leadership was not going to be convinced of the value of adding community care services to the system without evidence, but what kind of evidence was needed? Could these projects meet the test of "the business case"—i.e., spending money on them would either save more money somewhere else or would meet some other critical health plan objective? Could they meet traditional medical outcomes tests—i.e., to extend life, reduce illness, or improve functioning? Would medical and health plan leaders accept other "clinical" outcomes as worthwhile—e.g., home-bound members reporting less isolation, fewer frail members having to wear dirty clothes, fewer caregivers reporting stress? And even if any of these outcomes could be hypothesized, would it be better to have a few projects with control groups and extensive data, or many projects with weaker designs? The final section of the chapter explains the evaluation model that was devised.

KAISER PERMANENTE ELDERCARE INITIATIVES

Kaiser Permanente's audacious decision to leap feet-first into the potential quagmire of coordinating services for the frail elderly makes sense only in the light of the health plan's long tradition of innovation. Kaiser Permanente, after all, is not only the largest not-for-profit HMO in the world, it was also the *first* pre-paid group practice of any kind.

The concept of "pre-payment" was born in the depth of the Great Depression when a young surgeon named Sidney Garfield and an engineer-turned-insurance-agent named Harold Hatch came up with a radical idea for providing health care to the thousands of men involved in building the Los Angeles Aqueduct: The insurance companies would pay Garfield a fixed amount up front per enrolled worker, each of whom would pay a premium of five cents a day to cover whatever health care needs they might incur. The project proved so successful that, when the aqueduct was completed, Garfield was recruited by the famous industrialist Henry Kaiser to provide this new form of health coverage to the 6,500 workers and their families at the largest construction site in history—the Grand Coulee Dam. When World War II broke out, Kaiser again turned to Garfield to provide health care to the 30,000 workers who were building ships in the Kaiser shipyards in Richmond, California. After the war, both Garfield and Kaiser wanted to continue this new form of health care delivery, and, on October 1, 1945, the Permanente Health Plan officially opened to the public. Ten years and over 300,000 members later, the named was changed from Permanente to Kaiser Permanente, and the rest, as they say, is history.

Kaiser Permanente's effort to improve care for elderly members with disabilities may not be as dramatic or colorful as the story of its founding, but it stems from the same innovative spirit. It dates back at least to the 1960s, when the Northwest Region conducted a federal study to estimate the utilization and cost of Medicare's new home care and extended care (nursing facility) benefits (Hurtado, Greenlick et al., 1972). Congress had just passed the program but they had no data on what to expect. Kaiser Permanente's population-based managed care model gave it the capacity to quickly create, implement, and evaluate these benefits. The study showed that an extended care facility located adjacent to a hospital had the potential for improving rehabilitation and lowering costs compared to usual hospital-based care for these services. But, more importantly from an operational viewpoint, another finding of the same study changed the way KP provided care to its members. The findings from the home health aspect of that landmark study indicated that the Health Plan could add to the coverage of its younger members, the skilled home health service benefits that had become available to its Medicare members. While the cost of providing coverage for these benefits was not fully offset by cost savings in other elements of medical care, the net cost for covering these services amounted to pennies per month for the younger members. This was because such a small proportion of members used the services in any year. The addition of this coverage for the majority of its population allowed KP in Oregon (and later in all of the other regions of KP) to create a permanent skilled home health agency within the system, perhaps the first home health agency to be sited within an HMO.

In 1978 the Northwest region became one of the initial sites in the Medicare HMO demonstration of capitated payment and lock-in enrollment into HMOs for Medicare beneficiaries (Greenlick, Lamb et al., 1982). Prior to this, HMOs had to serve Medicare beneficiaries on a modified fee-for-service basis. The model eventually led to capitation payment for HMO services under the 1987 Tax Equity and Fiscal Responsibility Act (TEFRA), which later became Medicare+Choice.

Soon after the Medicare HMO demonstration, KPNW was chosen in 1982 as one of four sites for the Social HMO demonstration (Leutz, Greenberg et al., 1985). After the project received Congressional mandate in 1984, KP quickly enrolled its target of 6,000 new members, collecting high-quality data, and generally seeing its participation as a model for other KP regions and other HMOs (Greenlick, Nonnenkamp et al., 1988). The Social HMO experience was a source for key components of community care linkage that were drawn on by Manifesto projects, including screening the membership (Brody, Johnson et al., 1997), coordinating services for frail members (Abrahams, Capitman et al., 1989), and connecting community care to the medical system (Abrahams, Macko et al., 1992; Macko, Dunn et al., 1995). The Social HMO's other key feature—actually financing community care on an entitlement basis via special Medicare payments (Leutz, Greenlick et al., 1994)—was not an option for Manifesto sites since Congress had not yet decided on whether and how to expand the project.

In September 1987, the Kaiser Permanente Committee requested a study of services and benefits for the elderly. An inter-regional task force was convened to conduct the analysis, which focused on the long-term care needs of the elderly that lay outside the traditional scope of the program's coverage and services. Their report was submitted in December 1988, and the Interregional Committee on Aging (IRCOA) was formed in 1989. With support from the Garfield Memorial Fund (established with an initial contribution from Sidney Garfield to promote innovation in the KP system), the IRCOA was to guide a series of elder care initiatives over the next decade by bringing together regional chiefs of geriatrics, administrators, and researchers to digest and disseminate learning from these and other efforts. The IRCOA also organized a series of interregional geriatric institutes that brought together the health plan and outside experts to meet with hundreds of health plan staff. The IRCOA's Long-Term Care (LTC) Committee was the organizer of the Manifesto 2005 demonstration.

In 1990, IRCOA developed its Model of Care for older adults, which parallels the Social HMO demonstration in population screening, stratification, and detailed assessment for defined high-risk members and targeted interventions (including care coordination). The model was refined in a multi-region demonstration, and it was followed by a mandate to implement the model in all regions.

In 1992 the Garfield Memorial Fund supported the Center for Health Research in Portland to study whether high risk of disability could be predicted from Social HMO experience screening its members with a mailed, self-report health status form (HSF) (Brody, Johnson et al., 1997). A machine-readable HSF was developed for use by other KP regions, and the Screen Every Elder in Kaiser (SEEK) service was launched. In participating regions, the Center mailed the HSF to new elder members. When members returned the form to the Center, it was scanned, and population profiles and individual risk profiles were built and returned to site clinicians and managers, who used the information to reach out to members and build care plans.

The approach of the SEEK project received an impetus and an endorsement in 1997 when Congress made similar screening mandatory for new enrollees under Medicare+Choice. Since that time SEEK has surveyed 400,000 participants in 14 states. The SEEK system was recently formatted into a "frailty wheel," which allows quick and easy assessment of risk of frailty based on responses to four questions: age, needing assistance with medications, needing bathing assistance, and having health conditions that interfere with daily activities.

Another KP chronic illness initiative worth noting is the cooperative health care clinic (Beck, Scott et al., 1997). These clinics targeted high users of ambulatory clinic services. Members were asked to attend group visits with members who had similar conditions. Groups met monthly and, under the guidance of a health plan clinician (usually a nurse or social worker), set their own agendas for speakers and topics. Members were still offered the chance to meet their physicians after the group, but many found the groups a good substitute for visits. The clinics reduced emergency department use, visits to sub-specialists, and repeat hospital admissions. They also led to more visits to clinics and calls to nurses, fewer calls to physicians, and greater rates of flu shot and pneumonia vaccinations. Physicians were more satisfied with groups, as were the members.

In 1997 the Care Management Institute (CMI) was formed by the Permanente Federation to promote evidence-based medicine. The purpose of the CMI was to synthesize knowledge and identify best practices, then implement those protocols across the KP network with the express purpose of helping the various KP regions improve the quality of care and health outcomes for its members. From March through August, 1999, with help from the Garfield Memorial Fund, the CMI sponsored interregional work groups of interdisciplinary health care professionals to build on the work of IRCOA to develop a national population-based approach to eldercare that is tailored to the individual member. This group became known as the Kaiser Permanente Aging Network (KPAN).

The CMI's first eldercare product was the Elder Care Source Book, an eight-chapter manual for improving care. The sourcebook focused primarily on the health plan's main line of medical system practice with elders, but it recognized the importance of community care. Among its guiding principles for elder care, for example, were that "caregivers play a central role in the health of many older adults" and that "cooperation and collaboration with the existing aging network is critical." However, it was beyond the scope of the sourcebook to say how to create such aging networks or family linkages. The "transition module," for example, lauded family and community care connections but there were no specifics on how to connect, and there was no mention of what to do for members who do not have families. The nursing facility connections section did not extend to how to make connections with the growing number of frail members in assisted living and adult foster homes. The Manifesto 2005 demonstration attempted to fill these system and knowledge gaps by showing how to set up reliable linkages.

DEVELOPING THE COMMUNITY CARE DEMONSTRATION

Manifesto 2005 was developed in 1996 by KP program leadership, including a $3 million appropriation of health plan operating funds to conduct a demonstration. Citing demographic and medical practice changes that were creating larger numbers of persons with disabilities, the Manifesto posited that these changes could translate into market advantages for health plans that learned how to effectively address the needs of frail and disabled members. Yet the Manifesto recognized that appropriate medical services were only one piece of an effective strategy. Perhaps more important from the point of view of addressing unmet needs was community care, which the Manifesto proposed should become part of the health plan's basic clinical service package.

The Manifesto's notion of taking clinical responsibility for community care services did not mean that the health plan was committing to pay for them. Rather, the vision was that when a clinician or care manager saw a patient with disabilities, they should (a) be interested in whether and how needs for functional and social support were being met, (b) take steps to connect members with help if it was needed and wanted, and (c) keep tabs on what was happening, including communicating with community service providers. Clinical practice and benefits for prescription drugs were cited as an analog: even though health plan benefits did not pay for drugs for all members, clinicians would not think of practicing medicine without reviewing the need for drugs and prescribing them if indicated.

In September 1997 the LTC Committee of IRCOA met to begin planning the demonstration. The eight committee members drawn from all KP regions included physicians, nurses, administrators, and researchers, plus an outside evaluation consultant. Consistent with Manifesto 2005, the request for proposals drafted by the group stated that the purpose of the demonstration was to "fund proposals demonstrating new approaches to expand the program's scope of services to include a home-based and community-based services delivery system, not only for elderly members but for members of all ages who have need for expanded services." The Committee developed the following guidelines for getting the demonstration off the ground:

- Make the search for ideas as broad as possible by advertising the RFP in all regions through staff newsletters, email chains, letters to department chiefs, managers of clinical operations and continuing care services, letters to past Geriatric Institute participants, letters to the Garfield Memorial Fund mailing list, and word of mouth.
- Make the process of application as easy as possible by requiring only a one-page concept letter without a budget as the first response and a two-to-three page abstract for semi-finalists, and by giving finalists support from an LTC Committee mentor to develop full proposals.
- Primarily fund pilot projects and feasibility studies rather than controlled research designs. This was consistent with the path-breaking nature of the initiative and allowed more projects to be funded, especially new and practical ideas coming from clinical staff.

- Move quickly with an October 1997 RFP, concept letters due in November, abstracts due in January (1998), full proposals due in March, selection in April, a kick-off meeting in June, planning and staff hires in July-August, and operations beginning in August-December.

In the first stage, nearly 200 concept letters were received from all regions. The broad range of ideas and respondents constituted something of a key informants survey concerning issues facing members with disabilities and how those issues might be addressed. There were proposals to cover more services as benefits, to study needs, to link with a variety of community services, to manage care for high-risk groups (both in the community and within the HMO), and to make a variety of changes to strengthen how the medical care system worked in relation to the provision of office visits, nursing home support, mental health, post-acute care, and home health. Both the number of responses and the range of problem areas identified confirmed that service to members with disabilities was an area that needed attention.

After these letters were reviewed, a key decision was made: to focus only on service delivery and research projects that were outside the scope of the health plan's current medical care responsibilities. This criterion excluded many worthy improvements of home health, mental health, nursing facility, and primary care clinic services for members with disabilities. Also excluded were proposals for extensions of the model-of-care concept. While the need for these projects was acknowledged, it was decided that there had been and would be other initiatives to improve care in these areas. In contrast, this was the only chance that expansion of community care services was likely to have. In short, the committee decided to invoke one of the "laws of integration" discussed in the last chapter: the one who integrates calls the tune. The committee knew that its priority was to develop linkage and coordination projects, and it chose to empower project leaders who shared that vision.

This experience made it easy to see how integration with community care could lose out in a medical care system. This is not the priority of most of the system day to day, and it's certainly not the priority of the most powerful professionals (i.e., doctors) or administrators. Even those who are most concerned with members with disabilities have a list of improvements in their own clinical area. Without an outside stimulus like the Manifesto and the demonstration, a medical system is not going to empower the small number of people within it who do see non-medical community care as a priority.

With these priorities in mind, three-page abstracts were requested from 75 of the 200 applicants. The abstracts had to include budget estimates and approval from a supervisor. When these proposals were reviewed, the LTC Committee decided to ask applicants who were interested in similar client groups or services to work together to create unified, multi-site projects.

Full proposals were requested from 45 sites, including seven multi-site projects to be created. Each project was linked with a consultant from the LTC Committee to help answer questions, to provide guidance on budget recommendations, and to coordinate multi-site efforts. Almost all the individual sites asked by the demonstration management team cooperated with related sites in developing common goals and procedures for multi-site tests of their original ideas.

Ultimately, 15 projects composed of 32 individual sites were funded. A 2-day kick-off meeting was held in Portland, Oregon in June 1998. The site leaders presented their projects; the plans for evaluation, data collection and reporting were described; and the group projects had a chance to meet. The chosen sites represented a range of models for learning about members with disabilities and for better connecting community care with the KP system of care. Most sites proposed to explore direct-service approaches, while a few focused on developing new information. Most were primarily for the elderly, but five addressed the needs of members under age 65.

The discussions of the projects in the next three chapters are organized to illustrate key themes that emerged about linking the medical care system with community care services. The themes are not unique to the few projects in each chapter, but this organization puts forth exemplars of the range of issues and approaches to each theme.

The first theme is the need to connect with community agencies in more serious ways than the typical "best practice" of having a list of agencies by service and location to hand to patients who may need community care. Chapter 3 presents and analyzes three demonstration projects that developed and tested much stronger, two-way connections. These are not the demonstrations' only projects that tried to better link with community care agencies, but they show the types of efforts involved, the payoffs that can result for members, as well as the challenges to maintaining effective linkages. The three projects dealt with:

- Referral and access to adult day care, personal care, and transportation providers
- A protocol to define roles for and linkages to adult day services
- Volunteer programs to provide social support and increase access.

The second theme is the need to learn more from members and their families about the impacts of their disabilities and how to get them help if they need it. Chapter 4 presents projects that made pro-active efforts to connect with members to improve their access to services. The projects dealt with three areas of service in three types of community living situations:

- Educational classes to better prepare family members to care for members with disabilities

- A care coordination model for members living in adult foster homes
- Coordination of community care for elders residing in naturally occurring retirement communities.

The third theme is the need to make changes within the medical care system itself. On one level the changes involve consciousness and engagement among clinicians and care managers—moving out of the "don't ask, don't tell" dynamic when it comes to talking with members about the impact of disabilities. On another level it may mean developing new services within the HMO as well as establishing information and communication systems that support linkage and coordination with community care settings. Chapter 5 analyzes four projects that illustrate these kinds of efforts:

- A post-diagnosis dementia protocol to coordinate the care of members and their families with the Alzheimers Association and other community care services
- Home care aides for members with temporary disabilities who do not qualify for skilled home health care
- Para-professional community health workers added to continuing care teams
- Easy access to adaptive technology and supportive equipment.

Finally, the four projects for younger members with disabilities are set apart in their own chapter. Even though the demonstration RFP sought projects addressing the needs of members of all ages, the review panel received few that were not focused on the aged. Perhaps the IRCOA name and network hampered effective outreach to staff working with infants, youth, and working-age adults with disabilities. Chapter 6 reviews the four non-aged projects that were funded. These projects show that the three themes that emerged in the projects for elders held true for younger members, but these projects also supported new approaches:

- Systems to link the health plan and community care for a newly enrolled SSI Medicaid population
- Procedures to link health plan pediatricians with community care agencies, schools, and family caregivers that help children with developmental disabilities
- Group and individual interviews of members with disabilities to understand their experiences accessing medical care and community care
- Analysis of administrative and clinical data systems to identify members with disabilities.

The 15 projects at 32 sites were funded for a total of $2.26 million. Their purposes, target populations, locations, and funding levels are summarized in Table 2.1. The funding for most sites was clearly modest, and most added

TABLE 2.1 Summary of Demonstration Site Goals, Targets, Locations and Funding

Name of project	Purpose	Population	Location(s)	Funding[b]
Connecting with community agencies:				
Continuing Care Program	Link members to adult day services, home attendants, and transportation	Frail elders with weak informal supports	San Francisco, CA	$88,366
Dementia Care	Improve post-diagnosis care for demential patients	Members with dementia and their families	Denver, CO[a]	$127,000
			San Diego, CA	$46,600
			Portland, OR	$46,600
			Sacramento, CA	$46,600
			San Francisco, CA	$46,600
			Honolulu, HI	$46,600
			Total	$360,000
Adult Day Services	Link KP with adult day care providers	Frail elders interested in ADS	Seattle, WA[a]	$100,800
			Oakland, CA	$39,600
			Los Angeles, CA	$39,600
			Total	$180,000
Connecting with members and their families:				
Caregiver training	Teach family members to be better caregivers	Families of KP members with disabilities	Rockville, MD[a]	$129,028
			Denver, CO	$98,829
			Honolulu, HI	$54,402
			Southern CA	$98,500
			Total	$251,731

(continued)

TABLE 2.1 Summary of Demonstration Site Goals, Targets, Locations and Funding (*Continued*)

Name of project	Purpose	Population	Location(s)	Funding[b]
Adult foster homes	Improve out-patient care for members residing in AFHs	AFH residents and providers	Portland, OR	$51,080
Naturally occurring retirement communities (NORCs)	Help NORC residents set up supportive services networks	Residents of elderly high-rise coops and condos	Honolulu, HI	$100,000
Making changes within KP:				
Volunteers	Recruit and train volunteers to provide home- and community-based (HCB) supports	Frail and isolated elders in the community	Oakland, CA[a]	$84,000
			Anaheim, CA	$39,848
			Los Angeles, CA	$38,500
			San Diego, CA	$56,472
			Vallejo, CA	$60,000
			Denver, CO	$61,000
			Atlanta, GA	$60,180
			Total	$400,000
Temporary decline in functioning	Enhance in-home support through home health aides	Post-acute patient: who don't meet Medicare criteria	Honolulu, HI	$74,634
Community health workers	Enhance in-home support for through paraprofessional community aides	Frail members with weak informal support	San Diego, CA	$50,000
Adaptive technology (AT) and devices	Improve access to AT through referrals and display	Members who may benefit from an AT workup	Portland, OR	$50,000

TABLE 2.1 (*Continued*)

Name of project	Purpose	Population	Location(s)	Funding[b]
Serving younger members with disabilities:				
SSI Enrollment	Improve linkages between KP provider and Medicaid HCB services providers	SSI beneficiaries forced to join managed care	Vermont	$50,000
Early intervention	Link KP pediatrician with developmental services in state and local agencies	Children at risk due to established risks and delays in development	Cleveland, OH	$100,000
Voices of persons with disabilities	Focus groups & interviews about living and using services with a disability	Working-age members with disabilities and families of kids with disabilities	Denver, CO Portland, OR	$57,142 $115,895
			Total	$173,037
Disability event monitoring	Analyze data systems to develop ways to identify non-aged disabled	NA	Portland, OR San Diego, CA	$199,734
			Total Site Funding	$2,257,610

[a] Coordinating center for group project.
[b] Funding for most sites was cut 10% to 20% about 8 months into the Demonstration.

important in-kind services, space, and systems support to these funding levels. Another funding issue was that 15 months after the start of demonstration planning, and nine months after awards were made, the funding for the whole project was cut from $3 million to $2 million. Since the demonstration was funded from health plan operational funds rather than from the Garfield Memorial Fund, the project was vulnerable to cost cutting along with the rest of the operation when the health plan experienced high losses in 1998–1999. Sites were asked to find ways to cut their already slim budgets, and most found 10% to 20% to give. Since sites had already started their individual planning and development on the original budgets in Table 2.1, in some ways these are better reflections than the revised budgets of the level of support behind the projects' scope of work. This is not to say that the cuts did not affect the scope and achievements of the demonstration.

EVALUATING THE COMMUNITY CARE DEMONSTRATION

The community care demonstration explored a new idea: linking community care to a managed medical system across a range of populations and services. The new territory being explored—along with the limited funding available to any single project—meant that the demonstration was more akin to a series of reconnaissance missions than a coordinated set of scientific experiments. The LTC Committee decided that, rather than controlled designs, the proper evaluation model was to conduct feasibility studies focusing on the structure, process, and outputs of projects.

This kind of project provides information that is most usable for and most believable to the managers of medical care programs. Actually seeing a demonstration of a new approach to care is very convincing. And if the demonstration is organized in a manner that allows a fair approximation of the true cost of providing the service demonstrated; if staff are in place to actually deliver a new service; and if clinical champions emerge from the demonstration, the likelihood that the innovation will be adopted is increased greatly. While it is possible to have a great deal of confidence in the knowledge that is derived from randomized clinical trials, it is very hard to beat the existential knowledge that comes from actually implementing an innovation within a live health care system and watching it bloom in situ.

In the RFP and later instructions for proposals, the LTC Committee advised applicants that projects were not required to hypothesize or test impacts on patient health status or on health services utilization or costs. It was clear from reviewing early proposals that the interventions were not sufficiently defined and that the numbers of participants were too small to be able to demonstrate such results. It was even difficult to hypothesize that some projects would have these types of impacts. A few projects—particularly the groups—did ask outcome and impact questions, but most questions raised by projects concerned satisfaction and learning rather than impact on utilization, health status, or costs.

Each project had its own particular set of research questions, and answering these contributed to answering the overall question being addressed in the demonstration: What approaches can an organized health care system use to better understand the needs and wants of its members with disabilities and to more effectively connect them to community care supports? The overall evaluation was also interested in other general questions, including:

- How many HMO members had particular disabilities, what were their needs, and how could these members be identified?
- What were the range of community care services these members used?
- How could HMO staff coordinate with and support community care providers, including informal caregivers?
- What were the costs, benefits, and barriers to extending health system activities into community care services?
- How could successful projects be sustained and replicated?

These overall questions are addressed in Chapters 7 and 8.

Although the demonstration for the most part did not use controlled research designs, it did gather data on common elements, including quarterly reports on operational progress and problems, baseline data on participants, and aggregate utilization data on the services provided. Some of the group sites also conducted more detailed statistical analysis of selected questions.

The core process data were collected in quarterly and final reports from each site. Sites were asked to describe their major project activities, goals accomplished, barriers encountered, and how barriers were addressed. Project leaders also were asked to reflect on what key groups (members, community care providers, health plan providers and administrators, caregivers, volunteers) were looking for from the health plan and whether they were getting it.

In addition to process data, each project serving members administered a common Health Status Form (HSF) to collect a core set of health status and demographic data on participants. In most sites the respondents were the members with disabilities who received the services, but in some sites there were also other respondents (e.g., caregivers). The HSF data items were drawn from the KP Senior Advantage screening form used in most regions to screen new members over age 65. Table 2.2 lists the 25 required items. Most sites used the exact wording and formats from the Senior Advantage form, but there were exceptions for sites serving non-aged populations, since some of the items and question wording from the Senior Advantage form

TABLE 2.2   Core Data Items Selected from Senior Advantage Screening Form

Self-rated health	Helpers with ADLs and IADLs
Special treatments	Mobility outside the home
Health conditions	Special equipment use
Prescription drugs	Use of community care services
Conditions' impacts on activities	Current living arrangement
Inside mobility	Current housing type
Recent hospitalization	Current marital status
Recent psychiatric care	Race
Recent emergency room use	Hispanic origin
Recent doctor use	Gender
Recent nursing home use	Education
Help with ADLs	Employment status
Help with IADLs	

were not appropriate. Another exception to the core items was that sites did not need to collect items that were already collected from participants through existing data collection and reporting systems.

The HSF was designed to be administered by mail, but other approaches that fit better into the flow of a site's operation were accepted. At some sites the questions were part of face-to-face "intake" interview. At others they were administered as a telephone survey. To ease the barriers to entry for participants, a few sites were also given permission to reduce the number of questions. Several projects used the full Senior Advantage form in its machine-readable format, allowing the results to be quickly processed at the KP Center for Health Research in Portland at minimal cost taking full advantage of economies of scale and the continuous Medicare member survey processes.

In addition to the core process and HSF data collection, many sites did special studies. Most group sites assessed at least some aspects of their impacts on participants, including overall satisfaction with project services and pre-post differences in areas such as learning through project services and changes in community care service use. A few of the larger sites had sufficient sample sizes to explore questions about differential impacts by participant characteristics or by individual site in group projects. Some of these studies have already been published or submitted to peer-reviewed journals, and their general findings are reported in the chapters that follow.

Two projects did not serve or link members with community care services but rather collected and analyzed data to help the system better understand how to serve members with disabilities. One project explored whether it was feasible (and useful) to tap into the health plan's vast pool of administrative and clinical data to identify and characterize members who might have disabilities. A second two-site project used focus groups and in-depth, qualitative interviews with individuals to increase understanding of disabled members' experiences in accessing services—both within the health plan and in the community.

Once the intervention, data collection, and analysis plans were complete, each site had to seek approval of its regional Institutional Review Board (IRB). In several cases this turned out to be more time-consuming than anticipated. Some reviewers questioned the worth of the projects on the grounds that they lacked comparison group designs. Others required consent forms from participants, even when the only "intervention" was classes or gathering information and making a referral. In other regions, the IRB agreed that its local project did not require IRB approval at all. Eventually, all sites were either accepted or exempted.

The evaluation team was composed of an evaluation director (a university-based consultant), five internal research experts from the KP system, and a data center to collect and process HSF data. Under the direction of the principal investigator, the evaluation director was responsible for specifying the research questions to be addressed, defining data sets and data collection, analyzing findings, and preparing overall project reports. The data center documented sites' plans for collecting HSF data, collected and processed HSF data, and produced descriptive reports on demonstration participants as requested by members of the evaluation team.

The five internal experts reviewed the overall evaluation design, represented the evaluation to assigned projects in their geographic and substantive areas, and coordinated with their sites' LTC Committee liaisons. Plans for mid-way and end-of-project site visits by evaluation team members were dropped when budgets were cut.

SUMMARY

Kaiser Permanente has the good fortune to have the history, size, and structure that promote innovation and learning about how to keep populations healthy. Its core business is medical care—doctors, hospitals, nurses, medical social workers, therapists, and others—who deliver care within the confines of what is covered by traditional health insurance. Basing providers in large health centers allows the health plan to offer clinicians and members special supports that are impractical for smaller medical groups and independent practitioners to provide. These include the health plan's geriatricians, continuing care nurses, social workers, hospital discharge planners, and home health nurses. Although they are based in the medical system, these providers are particularly well placed to see where the medical system ends and what problems frail members face as they cross the borders into community care. Finally, having inter-regional research, professional, and administrative structures allows the health plan to raise issues and take action across the system.

On paper, the linkage and coordination projects chosen and shaped by the LTC Committee seemed responsive to the Manifesto 2005 call for developing a system of community care services for all of the health plan's frail and disabled members. Taken as a whole, the projects were broadly based in terms of targeting, they seemed to require little new financing for services, and at least the multi-site projects were charged to accommodate regional variations. They were also often logical extensions of the health plan's prior and ongoing efforts to improve services for elders, including the experiments to create home health benefits, the expansions of community care benefits and linkages in the Social HMO, case management and screening in the model of care, and the call to work more closely with caregivers and community providers in the CMI sourcebook.

The LTC Committee was also successful in distributing the RFP broadly and in eliciting practical proposals from grass-roots practitioners. Based on their insight and experience with everyday challenges, they proposed small but seemingly feasible changes to and extensions of what they were already trying to do. These were not projects dreamed up by academics or sophisticated health services researchers, and the LTC Committee and evaluation team did not try to recast them. The projects that were accepted did not by any means address every problem in community services for members with disabilities. From the proposals that were not accepted it was clear that there were many more problems. But the 15 projects and 32 sites were a good start. Funding for almost all individual sites was very lean, but the LTC Committee decided to make affordability one test of practicality; expensive improvements in services were not likely to survive even if they showed promising results.

The evaluation also followed the lean and eclectic route. It laid down a core procedure for collecting process and participant data, but it was forced to rely on the individual sites to collect the data and report their experiences. The few outcome studies were supported and directed by the multi-site teams. The chapters that follow show that the system worked better at some sites than at others, and together the failures and successes provide a strong overview of the problems, results, and promising next steps.

Beyond these general thoughts about the context and meaning of the demonstration, there are numerous specific questions that should be asked and answered.

- Which projects were successful and which were not, and why?
- What did community care agencies think of the the health plan effort,

particularly the KP vision of their services as part of the health plan's clinical concerns?

- How did members react? Did they have overwhelming demands that could not be met, or were the offered services greeted with little demand?
- How did health plan clinicians and managers react? Were the initiators able to get the attention and cooperation of physicians, and if not, were there ways to succeed without them?
- Was it a sensible idea to include younger members, or were their issues of a different order calling for different approaches?
- Are there any lessons beyond the success and failure of individual projects—that is, is there a synthesis of the experience that points to new linkage models to be tested?

The lessons are relevant not only to KP but also to other HMOs and the larger health care system. There are many compelling reasons why organized health care systems should consider fostering the inclusion of community care: The need is huge; families may be coordinating care for multiple elders and need streamlined contact points; the medical care labor force is shrinking and needs more partners; and persons doing hands on daily care in the community can be eyes and ears to monitor predictable symptoms and geriatric syndromes. Kaiser Permanente is special in its willingness and capacity to undertake a large demonstration like this on its own, and its health center system of primary and preventive care gives it an infrastructure of staff and information systems that are unusual in U.S. health care. Yet there are analogous staffs and systems in many other HMOs, as well as in consolidated sub-sectors of the medical care system (e.g., hospital systems with affiliated physicians and post-acute providers). And the more unified acute care systems of countries with universal insurance or delivery systems for medical care have much the same capacity.

The responses of community care agencies and family caregivers to the KP initiative also hold lessons for medical care systems more generally. The KP demonstration took place in eight states, and linkages were formed with a very wide range of formal and informal providers. Although there is truth in the statement that "all linkage is local," there are also general themes about the roles and capabilities of these agencies and the challenges they face.

REFERENCES

Abrahams, R., Capitman, J. A., et al. (1989). Variations in care planning in the Social/HMO: A qualitative study. *Gerontologist, 29*(16), 725–736.

Abrahams, R., Macko, P., et al. (1992). Across the great divide: Integrating acute, post-acute, and long-term care. *Journal of Case Management, 1*(4), 124–134.

Batavia, A. I. (1993). Health care reform and people with disabilities. *Health Affairs* (Spring), 40–56.

Beck, A., Scott, J., et al. (1997). A randomized trial of group outpatient visits for chronically ill older HMO members: The cooperative health care clinic. *Journal of the American Geriatrics Society, 45*(5), 543–549.

Brody, K., Johnson, R. E., et al. (1997). Evaluation of a self-report screening instrument to predict frailty outcomes in aging populations. *The Gerontologist, 37*(2), 182–191.

Greenlick, M., Lamb, S., et al. (1982). A successful Medicare prospective payment demonstration. *Health Care Financing Review, 4*(4).

Greenlick, M. R., Nonnenkamp, L., et al. (1988). The S/HMO demonstration: Policy implications for long term care in HMOs. *Pride Institute Journal, 7*(3), 15–24.

Hurtado, A., Greenlick, M., et al. (1972). The utilization ad cost of home care and extended care facility services in a comprehensive prepaid group practice program. *Medical Care, 10*(1), 8–16.

Leutz, W., Greenlick, M., et al. (1994). Integrating acute and long-term care. *Health Affairs* (Fall).

Leutz, W. N., Greenberg, J. N., et al. (1985). *Changing health care for an aging society: Planning for the social health maintenance organization.* Lexington, MA: Lexington Books.

Macko, P., Dunn, S., et al. (1995). The Social HMOs: Meeting the challenge of integrated team coordination. *Journal of Case Management* (Fall).

3

Reaching Out and Linking Up

Walter Leutz, Michelle Hillier, Enid Hunkeler, and Hanh Nguyen

T his chapter begins a four-chapter sequence that analyzes the individual projects in the demonstration. The chapters (and the projects within them) are organized to highlight three specific pieces of more coordinated systems of care: community care services, member and family needs, and the medical system itself. There is also a separate chapter for projects serving non-aged members with disabilities, and these projects review and enrich the same themes.

These topical separations of the chapters and projects are somewhat artificial, however, since almost all projects dealt with two basic questions: How do we get from here (fragmented systems of medical and community care) to there (linked and coordinated systems)? Project leaders also found two underlying questions more difficult and perhaps more important to answer: First, are these "our" problems (i.e., the medical system's), and, second, if they are, what are the paybacks for us and our members for addressing them? The second part of the question raises outcome and cost-effectiveness issues that the pilot projects can answer in suggestive but not definitive ways. The first part about who is responsible for rectifying the apparent separation is a better place to start.

Since it's an underlying premise of this book that there has historically been a separation between medical and community care, a useful preface to the discussion of the specific projects is to elaborate this point. Figure 3.1 dramatizes the issue. This picture was drawn by a community agency staffer at an outreach meeting to show how a small agency feels when relating to a large HMO such as KP. From the point of view of many community care

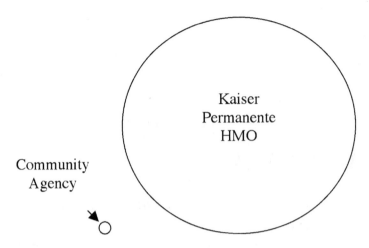

FIGURE 3.1   View of Kaiser Permanente from a community agency's perspective.

agencies, KP is a large, faceless, powerful, professionalized, and ultimately confusing system.[1] Ironically, if there were many more small circles, the figure would also illustrate how many HMO staffs view community agencies: small, weak, numerous, and hard to tell apart or really understand. From this perspective, KP is a specific case of a more general face medical care shows to community care and vice versa.

The disparities, separation, and lack of understanding would not be a problem, except for the fact that these service systems share clients. As things stand now, it's up to the clients and their families to bridge the gulf from medical care into community care, and this is a lot to ask. Community care agencies are no less confusing to members than they are to medical care staff. Newly disabled individuals and their families are unlikely to have experience with the range of services, the terminology, the eligibility criteria, the application processes, or whether there are sources that may pay for care. The members who need these services are generally the least able to figure out and coordinate the eligibility maze.

Nor are community agencies in a good position to know when patients from the medical care system are referred to them, or to know what's happening in the medical care of their clients. Where medical care benefits and services leave off is where these agencies often pick up, but this does not make it a smooth hand-off across system borders. The idea of better linkage is based on the notion that it would be valuable for these agencies to know

---

[1] Rural areas with simpler systems and more personalized relationships may be an exception.

more about who is coming across the border, what they bring in terms of services and benefits, what they are getting on the other side, and how to communicate with professionals on the other side.

These next few chapters will provide a variety of qualitative and quantitative evidence for why medical care systems should care about better connections with community care. The developers and the goals of their projects are described—their planning, development, and implementation experiences, and their results in terms who was served and how well. The projects show that there is value out there in the community for both members and health plans, and they show how this value can be accessed.

This chapter focuses on linking with community care for elders—what exists in terms of resources and how better connections to those resources can be made. The first project presented was a referral system proposed by the Community Based Medicine subdivision of the Department of Medicine in San Francisco—an ideal site to start the discussion. CBM has a long-standing role as the unit in KP's San Francisco region that handles post-acute care. While CBM's primary placement responsibility is Medicare-covered home health and nursing facility care, the unit also helps with referrals to non-covered community care, including the attendant care, adult day services, and transportation supports that were the focus of the project. The CBM's long-standing difficulties linking frail members with these services were the motivation for this project.

The second project was a multi-site effort to link with adult day services (ADS) programs. According to its providers and other proponents, ADS—alternatively called adult day health care, adult day care, and day center services—is a uniquely valuable service for many frail elders and other adults with functional and cognitive limitations. Participants are transported to a central place for a range of helping services (therapies, meals, bathing) and socialization for participants, and respite for family caregivers. ADS models range from social-model programs that provide mostly socialization and activities for less disabled and medically at-risk participants, to programs specializing in dementia, to medical-model programs that provide a full range of skilled and personal care services. Specifics vary by community and sponsor, and the availability of state funding through Medicaid is often a determinant of the scope and nature of ADS available in a community.

The third project connected with another type of community resource—volunteer services. The lure of volunteers—as extra resources, community builders, and for public relations—is substantial to community-oriented health care organizations such as KP. But any organization that has created successful volunteer programs knows that finding, using, and maintaining these "free" resources requires a substantial commitment of staff time and other resources. The quality of volunteer help is often worth the effort, however. Volunteers may be able to provide things that are difficult to buy—for instance, flexible transportation, a caring person whose time is not limited by the need to see other patients. Volunteers create relationships with the people they help that are unlike professional connections, and this is often just the type of social ties that isolated frail elders need. Whether to "grow your own" volunteers or partner with existing community agencies with volunteers was another issue, and the sites in this project took different courses.

These are not the only demonstration projects that reached out to community agencies—indeed, most did—but they are our best examples to illustrate the range of issues involved. The next chapter presents projects that highlight members and families—the issues they face coping with chronic illness and disabilities, and their experiences getting help. The third chapter in the sequence focuses on projects that illustrate issues inside medical care—how it now falls short in connecting elders with community care and how to make improvements. These three chapters thus build the three-sided puzzle that knits community, member, and health plan into closer patterns of care. By the end of these three chapters, a more complete picture of the structures and processes of linkage and coordination should emerge.

THE SAN FRANCISCO REFERRAL SYSTEM

The Developers and Their Goals

The nurses and social workers who staffed KP San Francisco's community-based medicine program had long-standing difficulties making successful referrals to community agencies. The goal of their demonstration project was to improve linkage with three key services—in-home attendant care, adult day services (ADS), and transportation. Improved linkages were intended to smooth access for health plan members, increase utilization of these services, and also improve care on both ends by supporting the sharing of clinical and service information. Another goal was to negotiate discounts for health plan members.

Planning, Development, and Implementation

The project coordinator received a supportive response when she approached community care agencies about the project. Although it was difficult to negotiate cut-rate fees, agencies were pleased to tell more about their services and to find out how to work more closely with the health plan. Besides meeting with individual agencies, the coordinator attended meetings in the community where information about new services and programs was shared. Having a health plan representative at these meetings was noted and appreciated.

The development process identified networks in which the coordinator or her staff participated to keep up-to-date on service system changes. They also obtained application forms and procedures, eligibility criteria, and charging information from the participating community agencies. They also asked agency staff about their experiences working with KP and other big HMOs. The agencies' biggest issue was how to work with the health plan when they had a problem with a member. Phone calls to KP went through a "call center," where callers often experienced long holds, and after the hold, the person taking the call often could not answer the question. The project's solution to this was a establish a single point of contact for community care agencies in the person of the coordinator.

Systems Learning

Through these contacts the coordinator gained the knowledge and skills to make more effective referrals. For example, by attending meetings of the Attendant Care Task Force, the coordinator learned that San Francisco was working to increase wages and benefits of attendants, which was putting many private agencies out of business and making it prohibitively expensive for moderate-income users to pay privately. The city was at the same time working on new subsidies for some near-poor and an employment agency approach for those who could pay. At these meetings the coordinator also learned that the California home attendant program had a new eligibility category just above Medicaid that some members could use to get personal care attendants. Attending a community networking meeting was the only way to get this information. It would be difficult for an HMO (and nearly impossible for individual members) to keep up with such changes without a coordinator.

Similar useful detail was gained by networking with transportation and ADS providers. For example, the coordinator learned that health plan members would be much more likely to qualify for the public para-transit system if their application listed functional disabilities rather than medical-diagnosis-related disabilities. She learned that one ADS center thought KP had been "dumping" difficult patients, and wanted to stop accepting health plan members, but communication about what an HMO can and cannot do cleared this up.

The contacts also uncovered opportunities for service substitution and coordination. The Bay Area ADS network offered training to their providers, which was also open to community professionals. When a KP home health nurse attended one of these meetings, she came back excited and enthusiastic, having learned that the ADS providers could do tube feedings and insulin injections. The kinds of advantages the single point of contact coordination provided were illustrated by the case of a member in ADS with a below-the-knee amputation. The day center wanted to know if he could learn how to use his prosthesis. The coordinator connected the agency with the KP physician and physical therapist, and this helped a decision about his treatment. Closer ties also helped the health plan and community care providers sort out who paid for what—e.g., mental health and foot care providers wondering what the health plan did and didn't pay for and how to bill for what they were providing.

Characteristics of Members Served

The project sought to serve 100 of 1,400 eligibles in the region during the 1-year test period. Table 3.1 shows that the 101 participants had many high risk characteristics. According to the health status form (HSF, administered in this site by phone), participants were predominantly female and widowed, divorced or separated. Thirty-one percent were non-White. Two-thirds needed help bathing, and nearly three-quarters needed help taking medications. More than half needed help with three or more ADLs, and nearly three-quarters needed help with seven of nine IADLs. More than half had an emergency room visit in the last six months; nearly all had health conditions that interfered with their daily activities; and 70% had four or more chronic health conditions.

Services Provided

The top half of Table 3.2 shows the success of the Referral Project in linking members to community care services. Data are based on a phone survey of participating members conducted near the end of the demonstration period. Clearly it was easier to link members to attendant care than to ADS: Of 101 respondents, 73% were still receiving either ADS (11%) or attendant care (58%) services or both (4%). Of those not deceased, only one-quarter had used ADS at some point, while 69% had used an attendant. Thirty-one percent had refused to follow through on their referral.

Participant Impact and Feedback

A sampling of member views of ADS gathered by the Referral Project (Box 3.1) shows why it was so difficult to get elders to use ADS. Resistance ranged from the seemingly simple act of getting there (not so simple for frail elders), to fear of new social situations, to cost. Those who did make the connection, however, were generally satisfied, as were the caregivers. Although attendant care was used more frequently than ADS, member's negative comments on the service were often in the same vein: not liking the attendant, high costs, and preferring a family caregiver.

TABLE 3.1 Participant Characteristics from Health Status Form

	Referral System (N = 101)	Adult Day Services (N = 210)	Volunteer Receivers (N = 159)
Health condition			
Self-rated health fair or poor	58%	60%	62%
Takes 5 or more prescription drugs	50%	28%	44%
Health conditions affect activities	96%	60%	69%
Severe memory problems	51%	34%	38%
One or more hospitalizations in last year	40%	44%	38%
One or more ER visits in last 6 months	54%	48%	38%
Reports 0-3 of 18 health conditions[a]	31%	57%	38%
Reports 4-5 of 18 health conditions	45%	23%	27%
Reports 6 or more of 18 health conditions	25%	20%	35%
ADL & IADL[b]			
Does not need help with ADLs	27%	16%	61%
Needs help with 1-2 ADLs	22%	32%	16%
Needs help with 3-5 ADLs	51%	52%	23%
Needs help with 0-3 IADLs	10%	22%	46%
Needs help with 4-6 IADLs	18%	17%	33%
Needs help with 7-8 IADLs	72%	60%	21%
Mobility			
Can walk up and down stairs	26%	32%	61%
Uses a wheelchair	39%	41%	36%
Equipment[c]			
Uses 0-2 of 10 items	61%	40%	60%
Uses 3-4 of 10 items	28%	43%	22%
Uses 5 or more of 10 items	12%	17%	18%
Living arrangements[d]			
Lives alone	39%	16%	57%
Lives with spouse	35%	32%	22%
Lives with child(ren) or other relative(s)	28%	27%	16%
Lives with non-relative(s)	14%	26%	5%
Current housing type			
My own residence . . .	88%	56%	81%
The residence of a friend . . .	7%	16%	7%
Group home, board and care, nursing home	5%	28%	12%
Current marital status			
Married	33%	40%	31%
Widowed, divorced, or separated	61%	57%	67%
Never married	5%	3%	3%

(continued)

TABLE 3.1   Participant Characteristics from Health Status Form
(Continued)

	Referral System (N = 101)	Adult Day Services (N = 210)	Volunteer Receivers (N = 159)
Race			
White	69%	74%	70%
Black or African American	19%	16%	21%
Asian or Pacific Islander	11%	6%	4%
Other	0%	3%	5%
(Hispanic origin)	4%	8%	3%
Female	69%	65%	80%

[a] Diabetes, high blood pressure, heart trouble, stroke, lung or breathing problems, chronic cough, cancer, circulation problems, stomach or bowel problems, urinary or bladder problems, arthritis or rheumatism, osteoporosis, hip fracture, Parkinson's disease, depression, severe memory problems, severe vision problems, severe hearing problems, other.

[b] ADLs include bathing including sponge, dressing, using the toilet, getting in/out of bed or chairs, and eating. IADLs include preparing meals, shopping for groceries etc., doing routine household tasks, managing money, doing laundry, taking medications, transportation, and using the telephone.

[c] Wheelchair, walker, cane, grab bars, bath bench, Hoyer lift, bedside commode, hospital bed, ramps, oxygen equipment, other.

[d] Referral project allowed multiple responses, which were made by 14 people.

BOX 3.1   Member and Caregiver Views of Adult Day Services
Transportation/getting there barriers
"Its too hard to get him up and dressed in the morning in time to get the bus."
"I can't get down the stairs."
Social situations/caregiver resistance
"He won't go without me and I'm not going."
"I'm too active and 'with it'—everyone else is worse than me."
High costs
"How am I going to pay for it?"
Program didn't meet needs
"I want 'real therapy'—not just exercise."
Caregiver satisfaction
"I can do errands when he is there for about three hours, or I can have lunch with a friend."

TABLE 3.2 Participation Rates and Reasons

	n	%
San Francisco Referral System		
Totals for all responses (n = 101)		
Attending ADS	11	11%
Has both ADS and attendant	4	4%
Quit ADS but has attendant	7	7%
Refused ADS but has attendant	11	11%
Attendant only	40	40%
Refused ADS and attendant	5	5%
Refused ADS	11	11%
Refused attendant	12	12%
Deceased	11	11%
Totals for live respondents (n = 90)		
Total using ADS	22	24%
Total using attendants	62	69%
Total refusing all referrals	28	31%
Adult Day Services		
Seattle/Tacoma (n = 15)		
Enrolled in ADS	4	27%
Entered nursing home	5	33%
Considering ADS	2 ·	13%
Not interested in ADS	1	7%
No response	3	20%
Oakland (n = 49)		
Enrolled in ADS	22	45%
Tried but quit	7	14%
Using attendant care instead	18	37%
Didn't get referral/waiting	12	24%
Los Angeles (n = 41)		
Enrolled in ADS	15	37%
Not enrolled: cost too high	12	24%
Not enrolled: cost and time/place	6	12%
Not enrolled: cost and transport	4	8%
Not enrolled: cost and home preference	4	8%

Provider Feedback

Box 3.2 shows mixed professional views of the Referral Project as a whole. Kaiser Permanente providers and case managers valued current information and personal contacts and reported increasing referrals to participating community agencies. Responses from directors of ADS centers appeared to reflect better linkages with some agencies than with others. The most frequent concern was having access to health plan information and providers when needed. Those who were happy got better connected; perhaps this was not the case for those who were less satisfied.

Summary

This project showed that community resource referral is a process, often requiring addressing social, emotional, and financial barriers on top of solving an immediate care problem. A well-connected, up-to-date, and persistent

---

**BOX 3.2   Kaiser Permanente and Community Agency Views
of Referral Project**

Kaiser Permanente Providers (11 responses, including 9 case managers)

"Updated information on a regular basis was invaluable, because it is always changing."

". . . helpful to have contact people at community agencies."

"I didn't get financial options for low-income, non-MediCal seniors."

"I use ADS much more often now."

"The project was great. It should have lasted longer and needs to be continued."

"A clear referral to a specific person in a specific agency with whom you have a relationship is much more likely to work the first time, and the first time is all the member may give to trying. This is part of preventive health care, since it allows members to be connected and getting their needs met before there is a crisis."

ADS Directors' reactions (5 agencies)

"It was difficult finding out who was responsible—I got a lot of 'not on my caseload.'"

"It improved service and shortened waiting time to receive physician reports back."

"Calling and being pushy is what helps. Being kind, patient and respectful gets you nowhere."

"Having a personal contact person made a huge difference."

staff network, such as the Referral Project developed, can shepherd members across the border into community care and keep in touch with what they are doing there. Without these efforts, HMO members are sent across with inadequate maps, few supports, and no reliable way to "phone home" to keep in touch.

ADULT DAY SERVICES

The Developers and Their Goals

The demonstration's three letters of intent to develop connections with ADS providers argued for the importance of this service to frail members. As with the San Francisco Referral Project, the lead staff of the ADS project was based primarily in continuing care departments or the equivalent. Working together, the three sites proposed a three-phase project. In order to begin to define the roles that ADS could play in the care for HMO members, the first goal was to learn more about ADS—e.g., the services provided, the types of clients served, how services were paid for. The next goal was to contact local ADS providers to work out what specific infrastructure would be required to better link members with providers. The last goal was to test the infrastructure and write a guide for other HMOs to link with ADS.

Two of the three demonstration sites were in California, a state that has an extensive network of large medical day care programs, which are reimbursed through Medicaid for eligibles. The Los Angeles site proposed partnering with three ADS providers and focusing on members with dementia, while the Oakland site wanted to work with the existing Adult Day Health Network and target members for any of the full range of appropriate needs. At the Seattle/Tacoma site, KP's Group Health Cooperative affiliate, two primary care clinics partnered with ADS. One clinic proposed linking with a local ADS provider with five separate sites, and the other worked with an ADS site that was in the Group Health therapy building next to the medical center where the target primary care team worked.

Planning, Development, and Implementation

While the three sites worked together to build pictures of the characteristics of ADS models in general, each met with its local ADS programs to learn in detail about their specific structure, operations, and clientele. The Los Angeles site used existing HSF screening information to try to locate ADS participants, while the other two sites sent the HSF to members who were already participating in ADS. Part of the process was to develop profiles of ADS users for education purposes. Joe M.—a member of one of the projects—is a good example of a good fit with ADS.

Profile of an Adult Day Services User

Joe M. is an 80-year-old man who lives with his caregiving wife. He has been diagnosed with Parkinson's Disease, atrial fibrillation, edema in the legs, and dementia. Joe has had two coronary bypass surgeries. Recently his wife has reported a noticeable increase in his short-term memory loss and also a loss of appetite.

Because of the difficulty of caring for Joe, his wife greatly appreciates the respite she receives while he is at the adult day health center. He is given a supportive, safe environment to socialize with other clients and staff, and he's able to participate in mentally and physically stimulating activities. Joe insists on attending on Fridays to participate in his favorite activity: Spanish.

Because of his wandering, Joe wears an alarm-activating device that prevents him from leaving the building but allows him to walk in the hallways when he is restless. Nurses administer noon oral medications, provide routine foot care, and provide oversight for medication compliance and weight maintenance. Staff occasionally assist him with toileting, dressing, and cutting food at lunch. Joe also requires reassurance throughout the day, as well as verbal cues and directions. He also attends an occupational therapy group two days a week.

The development team used this background, survey, and client profile information to create a recommended linkage infrastructure, which was flexible to allow each site to apply the components to its situation. The six-part infrastructure (Box 3.3) was detailed in a replication guide. Because ADS is often misunderstood, the guide recommended extensive education for both providers and members. It also called for systems to first identify members who might benefit from ADS and then to track what happens if a referral is made. Finally, it emphasized the importance of having ADS leaders inside the HMO—both a day-to-day staff leader and an organizational champion who could sell the program to other clinical and administrative leaders.

Systems Learning

The Los Angeles site's implementation efforts show the type of work that was done. Their development efforts tapped a broad range of health plan staff, including the ADS pilot coordinator; social medicine social workers; discharge planners at the KP mental health facility and inpatient hospital wings; physicians from internal medicine, family practice, and neurology; and a MediCal (Medicaid) representative. Besides a dementia diagnosis, to be eligible, members had to have a consistent caregiver and not be a candidate for institutionalization.

BOX 3.3 Infrastructure for Linking with Adult Day Services Programs

- *Medical provider education:* Distribute written materials (brochures, pamphlets, etc.), send email with links to websites, and present at team meetings (include ADS staff).
- *Member screening:* Proactively identify members appropriate for ADS. A one-page screening tool for use by providers was developed and tested.
- *Member education:* Put articles in member publications, distribute brochures, go to health fairs, and get providers/staff to talk about ADS during medical visits.
- *Referral tracking system:* Include referral to, enrollment in, and discharge from adult day services in member's record or organizational tracking system.
- *Information sharing system:* Define how HMO and adult day program will share clinical information.
- *A "home" in the organization:* Make it someone's job to maintain up-to-date information about local ADS and to transmit it to staff who make ADS referrals.
- *A "champion" in the organization:* Recruit a well-placed leaders (preferably a physician) who can command respect and organizational resources.

Los Angeles project staff initially tried to locate current ADS users by extracting data from the HSF that the health plan already sent to all new senior members in the Southern California region. The screener asked if the member was using "adult day services." When staff contacted apparent users by phone, they found that most who said "yes" had not actually used day care. Asking KP continuing care staff which of their patients were already using ADS was not a reliable method for identifying users either. This was confirmed when the site coordinator asked the ADH programs for a listing of health plan members. When she gave each case manager the list of their members attending day health, almost all were surprised.

The Los Angeles site's ultimate approach to finding new prospects for ADS was to use the broad range of staff enlisted for planning to do individual outreach. When eligible members came into contact with a participating health plan staff member, they were assessed and given (with family participation) the ADS alternative to home care, board and care, or nursing home. The coordinator contacted the referred ADS provider to see if the family called. If the family had not called, the coordinator contacted the family to see why not.

If the family contacted the ADS provider, a tracking and information system kicked in. The medical correspondence office and physician were notified, and release forms were signed by the patient or caregiver to allow the

ADS to have access to medical information if needed. Participating agencies notified the coordinator to confirm enrollment and to notify them if there were care problems or if services ended. *Kaiser Permanente* notified ADS contacts of changes in medical conditions or needs. The social medicine department tracked this information.

Characteristics of Members Served

Besides surveying current KP member participants in ADS, the project collected screening data from members who were identified as good prospects for referral to ADS. The summary of screening data from these two groups in Table 3.1 shows that the ADS members' profiles were similar to members in this chapter's other two projects. They had the highest rates of hospitalization (44% in the past year). Two-thirds needed help taking medications; 72% needed help bathing; and 60% used three or more types of adaptive equipment. Chronic health conditions and ADL and IADL limitations were highly prevalent but somewhat lower than among Referral System participants. They were least likely to live alone or in their own residence, and more than a quarter lived in board and care homes, assisted living, or nursing facilities. There were few substantial differences among the three ADS sites on these and other measures.

Services Provided

Each site showed different patterns of success in linking members with ADS. During the seven-month test period at the Seattle/Tacoma site, 15 members were referred from the medical groups at the two Group Health clinics. The reasons for referral included functional impairment (73%), socialization (60%), respite (47%), and cognitive impairment (40%). Although members were pleased that Group Health Cooperative was working on this, at the end of the period, only four had enrolled in ADS, while five had entered nursing homes (see the bottom of Table 3.2). At the Oakland site there were 49 referrals to ADS, and their rates of enrollment were near double the Seattle/Tacoma results. At the Los Angeles site, 41 members were referred. Primary reasons were respite (85%), inability of the member to be left alone (10%), and socialization (5%). Fifteen of those referred enrolled, but almost all of them participated on a more limited basis than they wanted primarily due to high costs: Mean utilization was two days a week and no more than eight months.

Participant Impact and Feedback

Feedback from members and providers give some insight into these referral levels and take-up rates. The major barrier to joining ADS that was reported by members (or family) at all three sites was the high cost of services ($40 to $100 per day). The next most frequent barriers were getting to ADS (transport, managing stairs, getting up in the morning), and caregiver and member resistance (including not wanting outside help, resisting change, and not liking other frail people). Also reported were lack of knowledge/information and not meeting needs (not enough therapy, wrong time).

The members who were able to overcome the barriers appeared to be positive about ADS benefits. A survey of Group Health Cooperative participants and family members was overwhelmingly positive (Box 3.4). Oakland participants were also said to be happy, and several had increased their days from two or three to daily.

Provider Feedback

Feedback from health plan staff revealed some of the challenges ADS advocates need to overcome to increase HMO referrals. Group Health Cooperative staff were enthusiastic about the project but wanted to know who was appropriate for day care and who for home care. *Kaiser Permanente* staff in Oakland felt that there could have been more referrals if caregivers had consistently told physicians and other providers about their respite needs. Lack of follow-through and long wait lists were also problems for health plan staff and members. Continuing care nurses and home health social workers were good at using the paper tracking form, but discharge planners in hospitals and skilled nursing facilities were not. Because the form used was not in the electronic system, if a nursing facility discharge planner made a referral to ADS, there was no way for other elements of system to know it and vice

---

**BOX 3.4   Group Health Cooperative Member Comments
on Using Adult Day Services**

"I was home by myself while everyone was at work and I became depressed. Now I am able to exercise and be in a social atmosphere. I enjoy daily activities and having a purpose."

"The staff nurse takes my blood pressure weekly and weighs me monthly. She also practices speech therapy exercises with me. She reports to my family physician quarterly. This program has made a major contribution to my stroke recovery, to my improved ability to speak, to my physical mobility and social interactions. The staff and volunteers are professional and caring."

"Since the day program ended for my husband, boredom has been a major problem as has loneliness and isolation. The program filled a vital need for him—and for me."

versa. In Los Angeles, hospital discharge planners were reluctant to refer to ADS even after extensive education. They felt more comfortable with services with which they had a relationship.

ADS provider staff had their own views. They were surprised to see how complex it was to get a referral and information from Group Health Cooperative. Partners in Oakland reported not enough collaboration to overcome their frustration in accessing the KP system, but they were happy to have some help and frustrated to lose the demonstration. In Los Angles, not having more referrals connect was a frustration to both health plan and partner agency staff. Project and ADS staff reported that KP MediCal members could have used ADS with state payment before they joined KP but they lost this when they joined.

Summary

In summary, the reports from health plan providers, community agencies, and members reveal six major challenges to improving linkage with ADS providers.

Questions about the value of ADS: Despite training by ADS and project staff, health plan providers and service coordinators continued to ask for evidence of clear positive outcomes.

Lack of knowledge about ADS by KP members: Members and families resisted using ADS, in part because they did not understand it. Staff found that multiple discussions and direct exposure were needed.

Cost and eligibility: ADS was expensive, and many members either could not afford it out of pocket or did not qualify for public subsidies.

Credibility with ADS providers: Kaiser Permanente was requesting their support to improve linkages during the project, but it was clear to all that the KP commitment would end with the grant.

Challenges following up referrals: A key component of the model infrastructure was a referral tracking system, but only one site (Seattle/Tacoma) made progress integrating this project into the HMO's electronic system for tracking and coordinating care. Because of this, members often reported they were waiting for more information after a referral was made.

Locating health plan members using ADS: Because ADS use was not in the *health plan* information system, staff did not have a way to identify members who were already using ADS. The health screening form question about ADS use turned out to have weak validity.

No single point of contact in the health plan for ADS staff: Partner ADS programs consistently said how difficult it was to make smooth connections with the health plan about the care of their KP participants. Each site set up improvements in the regular system, but none created a single position that could provide the information and foster the actions that were needed.

The ADS project illustrated the challenges of linking with a niche community care service. While no community care service is for everyone, ADS is particularly challenging because of cost, transportation, user resistance, and referrer misunderstandings. Yet it is by most accounts a very valuable service for the frail elders who do connect. Later chapters will discuss how it could fit into a larger linkage model.

VOLUNTEERS TO PROMOTE SOCIAL SUPPORT AND ACCESS

The Developers and Their Goals

This demonstration received more proposals for volunteer development (seven) than for any other area of community care linkage. Five were from California (Los Angeles, San Diego, Orange County, Vallejo, Oakland), one was from Atlanta and the other from Denver. The development team asked the seven groups to form a single project under the leadership of the Division of Research (DOR) in Oakland. The DOR dropped out as a service site to meet budget constraints.

The goal of the project was to determine if volunteers could help frail and at-risk members in four areas: loneliness, quality of life, satisfaction with care, and the use of social support and health-related services. Mixes of approaches to using volunteers varied across sites. Almost all proposed to offer telephone reassurance, while fewer included monitoring, transportation, and home visiting for more direct support and respite. The evaluation was designed to see who benefited most from receipt of services and what types of services were most requested and accepted. There were also practical questions posed about recruiting, training, retaining, and supervising volunteers.

Planning, Development, and Implementation

The group spent the first 6 months in planning and development tasks, including crafting a vision statement (see below), writing a volunteer training manual, and refining common research procedures and instruments. An idea of the complexity of starting and running a volunteer program is provided by a sampling of topics from the training manual index: publicity, flow chart, volunteer recruitment and enrollment, training curriculum, community linkages, volunteer matching, benefits and worker's compensation, volunteer evaluation, volunteer termination, recipient enrollment and termination, and companion forms. Each site modified some elements of the manual for its local situation—for example, the specific approaches to targeting recipients, developing volunteers, and choosing what types of help to provide (Box 3.5).

BOX 3.5   Site Volunteer Program Models

Atlanta: Targeted most frail one-third of at-risk members identified on the HSF. Partnered with Atlanta African-American churches to get volunteers to offer telephone support to caregivers of African-American members.

Denver: Targeted members with any of seven chronic conditions for telephone reassurance. Found and trained own volunteers.

Vallejo: Targeted Hispanic members. Used community benefit funds to subcontract with two faith-based groups to recruit and manage volunteers, who provided help with chores, transportation, and caregiver respite services.

San Diego: Focused on members with dementia in conjunction with two other demonstration projects (caregiver training and community health workers). Recruited its own volunteers, who provided both in-home and telephonic services.

Los Angeles: Recruited volunteers broadly in the urban community setting. Provided mostly home visits.

Orange County: Recruited volunteers through two community partners (a home-delivered meals program and an interfaith program) and KP Volunteer Center. Provided both telephone support and home visits.

Volunteer project vision statement: For the chronically ill adult, the social and emotional support we provide will empower enrollees, reduce loneliness, and provide hope. The program will reduce depression, improve the quality of life, increase satisfaction with care, and increase use of social and health-related services. We will reduce isolation and loss of control by tailoring the delivery of volunteer services to the expressed needs and desires of the disabled.

The sites and the coordinating center worked to maintain a common intervention and data base with enough flexibility for each site to tailor the program as appropriate. All recipients were asked to provide basic intake and exit information as well as the HSF. A subset of participants at each site were tracked more closely as a research sample, who completed baseline pre-test and ending post-test questionnaires concerning satisfaction, quality of life, use of community services, and loneliness. A two-site pilot test of systems was held late in the development period.

The most challenging implementation issue at most sites was recruiting volunteers. Three sites negotiated with community agencies to use their existing volunteer programs, while the other three developed their own volunteer programs and recruitment procedures. In both models it was agreed that the training manual procedures would be followed, and in the case of partnerships with faith-based organizations, special provisions were developed to set out what volunteers could and could not do relative to talking about their religion. Different approaches also had to be worked out for how volunteers in community agencies communicated with the health care team. All sites felt that it was important to screen volunteers carefully because of the vulnerability of the health plan members they would serve.

Procedures for how to recruit members to receive volunteer services were also developed centrally. Site leaders reached key providers and care managers through meetings and written materials about how and why to ask for a volunteer. For example, the Los Angeles site recruited participants through the geriatric screening system, which assessed isolated and depressed elders. They also went to the Geriatric Services meeting and set up relationships for referrals from hospice and home health services. Orange County recipients were recruited from the KP Senior Care Connections program as well as from clients of the community partners (i.e., meals recipients and church members). Site staff also met monthly with the service area's geriatrician. In Vallejo, recruitment got a boost during the planning period when the project secured the internal co-sponsorship of Members Services, Vallejo's site director, and a group of clinicians working to improve the delivery of primary care services. The Adult Primary Care team for frail elderly (physicians, social workers, nurses, home health, hospice, health education, and pharmacists) agreed to help identity frail elders who could use home support.

Characteristics of Members Served

The characteristics of participants were determined in part by cross-site requirements that care receivers be able to articulate the kind of services they wanted, live in a safe area, be able to hear and hold a conversation, already receive services to meet basic needs elsewhere, be able to cooperate, and agree to services. During the 6-month intervention period, 287 recipients were asked to participate, 247 accepted the invitation, 41 dropped out or were for another reason not matched, and 206 were matched with a volunteer. The HSF data on 159 participants in Table 3.1 show that four of five recipients were women, two-thirds were widowed, divorced, or separated, and 57% were living alone. In general they were relatively independent compared to individuals served in other projects, but relatively high users of medical care services. Sixty-one percent had no ADL limitations and could walk up and down stairs, but 54% did need help with 4 to 8 IADLs. Sixty-nine percent had a health condition that affected their activities; 35% had 6 or more of 19 listed conditions; and 38% had been inpatients in the hospital in the last 12 months or the emergency department in the last six months. Thirty percent where non-white, including 21% African Americans. Only 3% were of Hispanic origin.

Services Provided

Over the course of the six-month intervention period, 160 volunteers were recruited, 144 were screened, 118 were trained, and 113 were matched with a total of 206 recipients. A summary of the numbers of volunteers and recipients who were matched at each site (the first two columns of numbers in Table 3.3) shows that three sites matched volunteers nearly one-on-one with recipients, while the other three generally had volunteers serving two or more recipients. The summary of the predominant pattern of services that participants received shows that Atlanta and Denver provided telephone support only; Orange County, Los Angeles, and San Diego provided a mix of phone and in-person support (home visits, caregiver respite, chores, and transportation), and Vallejo provided only in-person supports.

These figures on the types of services delivered understate the volume of services delivered—both because they are limited to the six-month intervention period (which all sites extended) and because they show just the typical service pattern, not the number of contacts. For example, in the 19 months of operations through May 2000, the Denver site's 10 volunteers made weekly calls to a total of 63 members (2,125 calls in all), with an average of 166 calls a month in early 2000. Similarly, when San Diego's reporting period was extended 6 months through the end of 1999, it enrolled 96 recipients. The 25 volunteers serving them specialized: five gave phone reassurance to 28 clients; seven gave limited respite to 21; nine made friendly visits to 17; and seven provided transportation to 30. So in San Diego, most volunteers gave just one type of service, and most members received just one type of service. In the last 9 months of 1999, the San Diego volunteers made 1,395 phone calls, gave 132 respites, visited 150 times, and gave 96 units of transportation. An estimated 1,970 volunteer services hours were provided. At the end of 1999, 57 recipients were still active.

Systems Learning

The most important systems issue in the project was volunteer recruitment. There were multiple changes in volunteers, recipients, and staff, due to family crises, school/work responsibilities, and personal illness. The sites that partnered with community volunteer programs did not have to manage recruitment, but the decentralized model posed paperwork and communication coordination and oversight problems. Sites that centralized volunteer recruitment within the health plan had an easier time in these areas.

Atlanta partnered with Reaching Out to Senior Adults (ROSA), a network of 28 interdenominational churches serving predominantly African American populations. The 28 volunteers recruited agreed to serve 6 months, but most stayed longer: Of the 28 KP members enrolled in the first 6 months of 1999, 21 were still active in March 2000.

TABLE 3.3 Number of Volunteers and Recipients, and Number of Recipients Receiving Specific Services

SITE	Recipients Matched	Telephone Support	Home Visits	Caregiver Respite	Chores & Transportation	Transportation
Orange County	25	13	16	0	0	0
Atlanta	28	28	0	0	0	0
Denver	27	27	0	0	0	0
Los Angeles	29	3	21	0	0	0
San Diego	80	28	17	21	0	30
Vallejo	17	0	0	8	17	0
Total	206	99	54	29	17	30

In Orange County, two consultants were hired to coordinate the volunteer efforts at the two community sites (Interfaith Volunteers and Senior Meals and Services), which were partners in the project. A personal invitation to activists in local programs was the most successful recruitment method, but posters, press releases, and other types of outreach were also used.

The Vallejo site's collaboration with two faith-based groups was aided by grants from the KP community benefit fund. Faith in Action, an interfaith coalition established to provide informal, non-medical support for the frail elders, the disabled, and their caregivers, received a grant of $18,000 to support expansion to a new part of Solano County. Volunteers were recruited from 14 affiliated congregations, KP retirees, KP members, and current hospital volunteers. Catholic Social Services, an elderly outreach program providing emotional support and information and referrals through telephone contacts and friendly visits for isolated seniors, received a smaller grant.

The three sites that developed their own volunteer programs had to work harder to find volunteers. During the development period, the Los Angeles site recruited volunteers by setting up a coalition of churches and community service agencies. In the process they encountered many local agencies that were themselves trying to recruit volunteers. The site also reached out to the Retired Senior Volunteer Program (RSVP), KP retirees, local civic organizations, and the UCLA Center on Aging. They also made broader appeals through public service announcements, press releases to 16 local periodicals, the KP employee newsletter, brochures and posters throughout the medical center, and presentations to senior civic and support groups. As the project start-up date approached, all this had yielded only 75 responses with requests for more information. Of these, only 13 were trained. Additionally, they found that health plan insurance covered KP members' care to KP members, but they had to buy volunteer insurance for interfaith volunteers.

San Diego had serious problems finding and retaining volunteers in the North County area, which is 29 miles from the only KP hospital in San Diego. Transportation was a major concern for frail elder members there, and the site sought to address it through volunteers. But volunteers from North County turned out to have their own transportation problems, as well as health problems and family crises. Volunteers from other parts of the service area were unwilling to travel to and from North County. The site had to scale down the program because of this.

Denver recruited 10 volunteers from the health plan membership to serve a total of 63 members from three KP facilities over the 19 months of operations for which data are available. In contrast to the other KP sites that recruited their own volunteers, Denver staff reported no recruitment problems, and that they could have recruited more volunteers if they had needed more. They concentrated on recruiting KP members rather than partnering with a community agency because they were concerned that the funds for a community contract would not be there after the demonstration project ended. Denver gave volunteers 13 hours of training to conduct telephone support from KP clinic offices. Job description of senior care coordinators' responsibilities to Caring Callers shows the extent of work with volunteers, including weekly monitoring, supervision and record keeping; monthly reporting; quarterly recognition; ongoing identification of potential recipients; participating in volunteer training; and identifying potential callers. Other sites had similar responsibilities, but in sites that used community partners to recruit and manage volunteers, some of these responsibilities fell on the partners. Denver maintained Caring Caller after the end of the demonstration and even added a fifth medical clinic.

The impact of the volunteer services on recipients were measured in the six-site evaluation conducted by the Division of Research (DOR), with additional support from a direct community benefit investment. At the time of this writing, results were still being analyzed. Process records show that Denver may have averted two medical emergencies. One volunteer caller reached an elder who had fallen and was severely dehydrated. The caller phoned the health clinic, and an ambulance was sent. Another caller reached a woman whose medications had run out. An emergency shipment was made. Vallejo found that having enough volunteers to meet needs was a constant challenge, but volunteers who served were dedicated. The would-be participants often faced long waits.

Four of the six sites (Denver, Atlanta, San Diego, and Vallejo) were able to continue their volunteer programs past the end of demonstration funding. San Diego reduced active recruitment by early 2000, but public access TV ads continued. Three candidates contacted the office in the first quarter; two were interviewed; and two additional volunteers were waiting to be trained. A total of 28 participants were still getting phone calls, and there was also limited respite, friendly visits, and transportation on an as-needed basis. The San Diego site had 17 active and 10 inactive volunteers (due to health problems, family crisis, or transportation problems). Vallejo continued until March 2000, when the remaining 21 participants were transferred to Faith in Action, supported in part with a grant from the KP Community Health Partnership. After the demonstration ended, Denver added two sites to the initial three, all of which continued offering services.

Summary

The volunteer project showed that volunteers can be recruited and trained, and can be very effective in providing emotional comfort and social support to older, functionally disabled adults with restricted mobility while facilitating increased access to both health plan and community services in general. Key organizational elements to success were a centralized plan, skilled staff, space for the program (including phones for volunteers), a budget, training, and administrative support from the health plan. For some sites, an organizational affiliation with an existing community organization increased efficacy and impact. Operationally, it was important to screen volunteers for motivation and commitment, to maintain high standards and expectations for volunteers, to train them in an ongoing way, to have a training manual, to link them quickly with clients, to be flexible in volunteer assignments, to recognize volunteers with awards and appreciation, and to use a supportive team approach. It was important to be clear with both volunteers and recipients on the boundaries of what volunteers could and could not do. It was also important to link volunteers to a senior care coordinator who could identify potential recipients and provide on-site support to volunteers. And finally, it's worth mention that the volunteer mentality of generosity was also present among the staff of these programs.

LESSONS FROM THE PROJECTS

Having examined just three of the 13 projects, firm lessons about how to improve connections with community care for members with disabilities cannot be drawn, even in the area of the primary focus for this chapter—community care agencies themselves. Nevertheless, these projects provide insight into the status of community care connections prior to the demonstration, the whys and the hows of improving connections, and the challenges to continued success. Even these modest projects required new thinking, new activities, and additional resources. Lessons begin with an assessment of where the system is and then move into how to change it.

Gaps in the Cultures of Care

The remedy to poor connections to community care appears to require more than convincing providers to spend more time talking to patients about community care needs and then making better referrals. As currently configured, medical care providers and case managers often not only do not understand community care agencies, they do not have confidence that community care will take care of their patients—at least not the same confidence they have when they refer to skilled care providers such as home health agencies.

The gulf between medical and community care agencies is not simply a matter of separation, it's also a matter of underlying differences in the ways the two sectors operate and think. For an HMO like KP, making a referral to the community care system is fundamentally different from making a referral to covered health plan services. When members are covered by Medicare, for example, eligibility criteria are known, coverage is generally assured, the agency receiving the referral has obligations to provide care in a timely manner, and the referral is entered into the health plan information system so other health plan providers know it was made and can follow up. For the health plan's established continuing care units, there are also established personal relationships with receiving agency staff.

In contrast, none of these supports to successful linkage apply to community care referrals. Staff members in the HMO generally work from a long list of small providers with varied services. Rather than staffers making the connection themselves, it is more typical that community care referrals are given to members, and the members are ultimately responsible for calling the community agency to obtain more information and set up the services. The lack of collaboration between the health plan and community agencies reduces the chances that the member's social and medical needs will be met.

Even if members do call, they are likely to be faced with high charges for private services, waiting lists for publicly funded services, and functional rather than medical eligibility criteria. On top of this, community care services provide help that is often personal and intimate, which would-be users have taken care of by themselves for most of their lives, and likely with the help of a family member as their capabilities have declined. All this leads to difficulties making smooth connections to helping services, even when most of their costs are covered as benefits, as in the Social HMO (Leutz, Capitman et al., 2001). Connecting with volunteer services does not pose cost barriers, but the other barriers about knowledge of where to go and how to connect apply, since volunteers are essentially supplements to more substantial formal or informal services.

The Linkage Advantage

Despite these challenges, the case studies in this chapter highlight reasons for health plans to work on improving community care connections. Knowing more about community agencies helps the medical system make more referrals and better referrals, and this translates directly into more help for members with disabilities and for their families. Community care agencies are numerous, local, changing, and distinctive in terms of eligibility and procedures. By keeping up on what's offered and who qualifies, better fits can be made, and this in turn increases the likelihood that the member will actually get help. By developing personal relationships with community agency staff and by establishing more explicit linkage arrangements and follow-up systems, hooking up is not left to the member. Closer relationships also hold promise of improving the quality and efficiency of care on both sides of the system. Knowing what's happening with the client's medical care can help a community agency avoid duplicating things like home support and therapy. Agencies and volunteers can also provide things like transportation to or interpretation at medical appointments. Finally, closer community agency and volunteer service ties can improve care within the health plan by letting health plan staffs know what's happening in the community and taking advantage of chances to improve communications and compliance (See chapter 4 for more on this).

Linkage Mechanics

These projects provide lessons in how to link. Three levels for action stand out: information, operations, and organization. Informational activities may include sharing and distributing brochures, training medical providers about service eligibility and application forms, creating space for community care agency participation in health fairs and open houses, and holding in-service training by community care staff for medical care providers and staff who lead linkage efforts. Operational mechanisms include creating a single point of contact or naming a dedicated staffer for community agencies and members to contact for information and action; establishing referral, follow up, and tracking procedures (preferably electronic and thus available to all providers); and joint protocols covering these and other issues. Organizational ties can strengthen the linkage at a long-term and strategic level. This includes actions such as medical staff service on community care agency boards, medical staff participation in community committees and task forces (which can spawn new linkages), sharing space for joint activities (e.g., offering caregiver training classes), negotiating special rate and access agreements, and supporting community agencies through community benefit funds.

All Linkage is Local (Almost)

The projects also show that these types of basic guidelines need to be tailored to the local situation in both the medical and community care systems. For example, the sites in the ADS and volunteer projects each worked together to develop common approaches and protocols for linkage. These were useful exercises for gaining knowledge, credibility and mutual support, and all sites followed the guidelines' basic cores. Implementation, however, was also a local matter, and it was necessary to create local relationships, to learn the strengths and weaknesses of local service systems, and to be able to incorporate the health plan's own local priorities.

The apparent differences in the ease of linking with adult day services providers and local volunteer services illustrates the uneven and varied nature of community care agencies. On the one hand, volunteer services were generally acceptable to members and free, but they were not always easy to find; members who wanted a volunteer often ended up waiting until one was available, in part because the project was new and funding was tight.

On the other hand, even though ADS providers were interested in collaboration, the success in getting members into ADS was uneven. Some sites had much higher rates of successful referrals, but all sites had seemingly low overall rates of connecting members with ADS. The differences in success rates also have to do with the fact that volunteer services (and a variety of other self-help/advocacy-based services) are generally free or low cost, while direct care services like ADS are relatively expensive.

Projects in chapters to come will repeat these patterns, highlighting the facts that community care services vary in availability, user fees, and secondary barriers (e.g., transportation). Medical care providers that want to connect with community care must be prepared for some frustration with the gaps in service, but they can also go beyond this and become allies to advocate for improvements in the system. Once again, there are state and national venues for this kind of advocacy, but much of the groundwork and education is a local affair. Having powerful medical allies advocating for community care—instead of, or at least in addition to, advocating for more resources for medical care—could be a real turning point in building an adequate system.

Willing but Cautious Partners

Of course, the success of the KP demonstration projects depended on the willingness of community agencies to cooperate. Fortunately, interest was seldom a barrier to any of the projects in the demonstration. Community agencies were eager to have closer relationships with the health plan and pleasantly surprised that the health plan was making the effort. Yet they were cautious—some had seen previous efforts to improve connections that later withered, others felt that they gave value to the health plan but received little in return, and others feared competition for resources, as in the case of KP's recruiting volunteers from the same pool as theirs. The types of givebacks that community agencies asked for included not only referrals but appropriate and well-made referrals, easy access to HMO staff and information regarding clients they were serving, clarity and even flexibility in HMO benefits related to their clients' community care needs (particularly regarding therapies and home health), political support in the form of serving on boards and participating in community planning, commitment to long-term relationships and, finally, material support for efforts that involve direct collaboration or special consideration for health plan members.

Challenges

While the projects had many successes, these three case studies also show that the models were usually easier to put together on paper than in practice.

Updating information and training new staffs were constant needs. Matching members who needed services with the eligibility criteria and financial support available for community agency services often blocked access. And maintaining gains after demonstration funds stopped supporting special staffs and systems was also a challenge.

In the San Francisco referral project, at the end of the demonstration period, the coordinator's position (a new position) was terminated. The three ADS sites were also scaled back at the end of grant support, but all maintained some features. Under the leadership of a "physician champion," the Seattle/Tacoma site planned to establish a database to track referral and enrollment in ADS (the only site to do so). In Oakland, ADS providers lost the single point of contact, but a nurse case manager agreed to be a contact if other routes did not work. In Los Angeles, staff members who had been educated agreed to continue to offer ADS to members. The KP staffer making the referral will need to track the referral, and partner ADS sites will log KP members. The six volunteer sites showed the best potential for continuation. Four continued to recruit, train, and match volunteers past the end of the demonstration. Factors helping continuation may have included the elan of the development team and the strong links established with the community partners.

These three projects—as well as the others to come—show that the demonstration's vision of linking and coordinating with community care is realistic but that it takes real work to achieve it and keep it. The community care system is more fragmented and less well funded than medical care, and systems vary greatly from community to community. Yet there are real and valuable resources there for members, and the two-way communication and cooperation embodied in successful linkage creates an infrastructure of support to help members and their families navigate across the divide and connect with help. The next two chapters take up two more angles to making connections work. The first focuses on members and families, and the next looks more closely at what needs to happen within medical care systems. Together, these three chapters lay out the pieces of the linkage and coordination model.

REFERENCES

Leutz, W., Capitaman, J., et al. (2001). A limited entitlement for community care: how members use services. *Journal of Aging and Social Policy, 12*(3), 43–64.

4

Individuals with Disabilities and Their Families: Who Are They and What Helps Them Connect with Services?

Walter Leutz, Alissa Au, Kathy Brody, Connie Keyes, Marna Flaherty-Robb, and Phillip Percy

W hy should medical care providers and insurers care about whether their patients and beneficiaries with chronic illness and disabilities need or use community care? Will it save them time or money? Help them do a better job? Make their customers more satisfied or improve their health status? Or is it just a nice thing to do that can be relegated to the long list of other things that would be nice to do but that are not among the first-order priorities that actually receive attention? Similarly, from the point of view of the community care system, what are the advantages of understanding the medical care plan and knowing the planners?

To continue exploring answers to these questions, this chapter peers into life in the community for people with disabilities. The answers are not very direct in terms of cause and effect: get an elder in day care, and hospital utilization will go down; open a channel between the doctor and a caregiver, and blood pressure gets controlled through compliance with medications. Perhaps these kinds of results can be achieved and proven someday when systems improve, and care plans include community services essential to the success of the medical care plan.

Rather, the focus here is on how to gain information and understanding about the lives of patients and clients with disabilities and to use it to help them access the resources to improve the quality of their lives. Individuals with disabilities live in communities, and they are well or poorly connected to resources there. If they have supportive families, they will have the advantage of extensive resources; if they do not, their potential support is much less. Similarly, financial resources matter—at the high end where services are affordable, at the low end where they may be free, and in the broad middle where expense matters. Individuals also have attitudes, needs, and preferences that affect their willingness and ability to ask for and get help. Understanding the community life space of patients outside the medical setting is more than collecting data—it's putting data and other knowledge together in ways that will allow medical care staff to understand the situation.

What is it about individuals' functioning, relationships, living spaces, resources, attitudes, and opportunities and barriers to using services that is important for the medical care system to know? Who in the system needs to know what? What are the ways to get information about community care options and access to individuals, and, in turn, what are the ways to get information from individuals about their community care needs? Finally, how can service access points and service options be designed to accommodate the variety of resources and preferences of would-be users?

Kaiser Permanente and other health plans know very little in a systematic way about who their functionally at-risk individuals are and what they need and want. Within modern health plans many ready-made sources of information are available about medical care diagnoses and utilization, but precious few contain information about cognitive and functional status or about individuals' living arrangements and coping strategies in the community. Getting these types of information requires new data collection; it requires thinking about what points of contact should be exploited to collect data; and it takes new collection tools.

There is also an issue about who needs to know what when. Few primary care physicians or specialists consistently and systematically ask about community care needs and support, even though in some cases they may know things anecdotally. What should they ask and why? What should be recorded for future reference and for use by others? Or should the systematic collection of these kinds of information be the responsibility of other staff? Sharing and gathering information is time-consuming for both members and staff, and repetition and collection of unused information is not only inefficient, it can be a barrier to access if members resist complying.

Medical care and community care also must have ways to communicate effectively with would-be service users about what support and services are actually available in the community. While KP and other health plans are used to communicating information to members, the content and targeting of community care linkage messages are distinct. A starting proposition about communication strategy may be that the approaches a health plan is already using to communicate about medical care and prevention issues may be largely transferable, but the particulars may need to be adapted and additional content added.

Finally, there are also things that it would be helpful to know in terms of what capabilities and resources each patient has (or lacks) to access community services, as well as what should and can be done to make it easier to connect to specific services. From the patient's point of view, what is it that makes it easy or difficult to connect to an information source, a referral service, or a direct source of help? Are there things that medical care can do to make the connection easier and the fit better? How can a medical system know if services offered are the ones that individuals want, who is well served, and who is left out and may need alternatives?

This chapter explores how KP tried to identify which members might use new community care service options, which members responded (according to demographic and health status data collected), and how the new arrangements worked out from the members' points of view. The three projects in this chapter provide three windows into the life spaces of members with disabilities. They also show alternate ways to reach out to and connect with members in different situations in order to provide information, service options, and, ultimately, help.

The first project approached frail members through their caregivers (almost always a family or "informal" caregiver) by offering workshops designed to improve skill, knowledge, and comfort with caregiving. Because of the rapidly aging U.S. society and the increase in numbers of persons of all ages with disabilities living at home, many family members take on the caregiving role. Helping caregivers has become a hot political topic (at least as hot as long-term care issues get in recent years) and a growing research interest, particularly since studies have shown high economic value of caregiving (Arno, Levine, et al., 1999), the economic cost of caregiving to women (Doty, Jackson, et al., 1998), and the impact of stressful caregiving on depression (Emanuel, Fairclough, et al., 2000) and mortality (Schulz & Beach, 1999).

The second project sought to improve linkages with members living in adult foster homes (AFH) in the Portland, Oregon area. Oregon AFH providers serve up to five dependent adults, making the AFH the smallest and most community-based of group residential alternatives to nursing homes—larger options being board and care homes and assisted living. The paid caregivers in AFHs are paraprofessionals, trained a minimum of 80 hours and licensed by the state to provide 24-hour care. Eighty-three percent of homes serve residents who need assistance with all ADLs but who are not dependent in more than three. At the time of the study, Multnomah County had about 600 AFHs, 59% single-home operations and 41% owned by operators with more than one home. In most of the single-home models, the owner is also the primary caregiver. In the multiple home operations, most caregivers are hired. Although AFH residents are nearly as dependent as nursing home residents, no regulations require regular primary care visits or nursing staffing. The motivation for this project was to better understand and address the health care quality issues these settings raise for a health plan with growing numbers of members residing there.

The third project aimed to assess needs and develop a supportive services system in several high-rise buildings in the Waikiki section of Honolulu. The project treated the buildings as "naturally occurring retirement communities" (NORCs)—that is, unplanned concentrations of increasingly disabled elders who are "aging in place" rather than moving to congregate settings like AFH, assisted living, or nursing homes. Callahan and Lanspery (1997), among others, have proposed policies and service models that respect the preferences of elders to remain in their homes and that take advantage of population density to increase efficiency of service delivery. Their "supportive service model" relates to frail elders as citizens of communities rather than as patients; it helps elders work with community agencies to organize services around their NORC rather than around the individuals in it.

These three projects were chosen to illustrate member and family themes because they highlight three distinct contextual issues: the presence of informal caregivers, the receipt of formal care in supportive housing, and the service opportunities and challenges posed in independent retirement apartments. The members served by other projects in the demonstration were often in one of these living situations; but to round out the picture, members living in their own homes or apartments in the broader community should be included. Frail elders are more likely to reside in particular places and living situations, but they also reside most anywhere. The trick for helping organizations is to know where they are, to understand what that means, and to create the supports that get them the help they need and want.

CAREGIVER TRAINING AND SUPPORT

The Developers and Their Goals

Letters of intent to develop caregiver training and support projects were submitted by five KP teams in four regions: Denver (2), Hawaii, Mid-Atlantic, and Riverside, CA. They were initially focused somewhat differently—e.g., on empowering care receivers to better manage relationships and resources, on reducing risk of depression for members and families, on caregiver training (2), and on member-centered self-help. When asked by the development team to pull together a single project, four were able to develop a common focus on caregiver training and education. The team interested in care receiver empowerment decided not to change its focus and ultimately was not funded.

The site development leaders included two social workers, a health educator, and a nurse. A nurse/administrator consultant from the demonstration planning team was also active. Their goals were to identify and connect to at-risk caregivers, to provide didactic and supportive training, to educate health plan staff about caregiving issues, and to evaluate implementation of the project and its success in reaching and helping caregivers.

The team proposed to use a curriculum developed by the Roslyn Carter Institute in Georgia (as initially proposed by one of the Denver teams). The Institute was pleased to see a broadening of the use of its training materials. The curriculum—*Caring for You, Caring for Me* (Haigler, Mims, et al., 1998)—consisted of five, 2-hour modules of group work that included presentations by a facilitator, large and small group interactions, and some role play. The five modules were

1. what it means to be a caregiver,
2. taking care of yourself,
3. building cooperative relationships,
4. preventing and solving problems, and
5. accessing and developing resources.

Planning, Development, and Implementation

Staff from the Carter Center worked with health plan staff to train the trainers and modify the curriculum for the KP setting. This included a two-and-a-half-day workshop in Denver attended by five leaders from all the sites, as well as 15 local caregivers.

During the eight-month development period, project staff also developed an extensive effort to find and refer caregivers to workshops. This included articles in KP and partner agency newsletters; flyers, brochures, and posters in KP and community partner sites; and in-service training for health plan providers and care coordinators about the workshops and how to refer caregivers. The communications efforts of the Denver site were extensive but not atypical (Box 4.1).

To coordinate information and enrollment, a caregiver support and referral phone line was set up at each site, where interested caregivers could leave their name, address, and phone number. The project protocol was that the phone line message would say that no one from the health plan would call back unless asked; rather, the phone line staff would mail meeting and enrollment information to callers. If the caregiver called back to enroll, a confirmation letter and map to the training site would be sent.

BOX 4.1   Denver Caregiver Outreach Activities

- fliers in all facilities at check-in, pharmacy, and on elevators
- note pads for physicians and staff to give to members
- ads in local publications
- education section in KP web site
- fliers to targeted staff (senior care coordinators, chronic special needs nurses, disease management nurses, alternate care staff)
- fliers to community agencies and ads in their newsletters
- two-color brochures to mental health, primary care, medical offices
- voice mail to staff at medical offices regarding initial programs
- easel-stand posters in medical offices with monthly programs scheduled
- Rx pads and descriptive letters to 600 providers and front desk personnel, optical departments, and chronic special needs nurses
- 7,000 fliers in medical offices during October flu clinics
- notice in weekly employee newsletter during caregivers week
- in-service with front desk supervisors
- public affairs feature story
- schedules of workshops listed in "community news" sections of local papers
- first quarter schedules to contracted providers (hospice, VNA, etc.)

If they had questions they would be instructed how to call to speak directly to a staff member. Workshops were free of charge to both KP and non-KP participants.

Each site offered workshops for at least 12 months. All four started out with the five-session format, but three changed to a three-session format when participants reported that it was difficult to attend that many sessions. One site also mailed the curriculum workbook and other printed and audiovisual resources to caregivers who could not attend the workshops.

Most of the workshops were led by KP staff at KP facilities, but when Colorado had a hard time recruiting internal people, they turned to the community, where they successfully partnered with the local Alzheimer's Association, Stroke Association, and Multiple Sclerosis Society. Kaiser Permanente Denver and the Alzheimer's Association also tied the caregiver workshops to the demonstration's dementia project. The Director of Education for the Alzheimer's Association took the training and ran one workshop, and the association agreed to mail out information about the workshops to people calling their help line.

At the first workshop session, caregivers were asked to complete the HSF for themselves (17 items) and a similar form for their care receiver (25 items). Participants were also asked at the first session to respond to a 10-item questionnaire. The first 8 items were a caregiver preparedness scale adapted from Archbold and Stewart (1992), which inquired how prepared they felt (on a four-item scale ranging from "very well" to "not at all") to handle a range of caring tasks. The ninth question, which inquired how much the caregiver "enjoyed spending time with the care receiver"—an indicator of the quality of the caregiver/care-receiver relationship—was added to the scale for some analyses. A tenth question asked whether they often felt depressed or sad. Participants were asked to complete the questionnaire again at their last session. The before and after scores to these scales were the primary outcome data for the project.

Besides these participant and outcome data, the sites also (a) logged the number of inquiries to the call-in line, (b) surveyed participants regarding satisfaction with the workshops, and (c) conducted telephone surveys with samples of non-participants. Interpretations of these data are also reported below. All sites also chose to journal specific activities, communications, and systems issues so that lessons could be ultimately brought to customizing the programs to meet members' expressed needs.

Services Provided

From 10/98–10/99, the four sites generated over 1,100 phone calls. About half of the callers (596) attended at least one workshop, and 428 attended at least two. Ninety-five percent were health plan members. The large majority of inquiries were handled by volunteers and administrative staff—i.e., sending workshop information by mail and scheduling and confirming participation. Professional backup staff received few requests for further help.

It took three to four months of lead time to generate enough referrals to hold workshops, and this was in large HMO settings. Recruiters found that an article in member newsletter was a good way to get a jump in referrals, but it was short-lived. For example, an article in a member newsletter mailed to 500,000 members created a jump of 80–100 names.

Characteristics of Members Served

Table 4.1 shows the characteristics of the 467 participating caregivers who completed the health status screener for themselves, as well as the data caregivers reported for 418 care receivers. The typical sample caregiver was female, White, married, and relatively healthy and independent in functioning. Other data not included in Table 4.1 show that 66% of the caregivers were living with the person receiving care, but only 40% were the spouse of the receiver; 30% were the children of the care receiver, 24% were another relative, and 6% were not related. Thirty-nine percent were college graduates, and 39% were employed outside the home. More than 50% had been providing care for three or more years, and 42% provided care for 40 or more hours a week.

TABLE 4.1 Participant Characteristics[a]

	Care Receivers (N = 418)	Care Givers (N = 467)	Adult Foster Homes[b] (N = 296)	NORCs[c] (N = 114)
Health condition				
Self-rated health fair or poor	64%	18%	61%	19%
Takes 5 or more prescription drugs	35%	na	37%	17%
Severe memory problems	29%	na	44%	0%
Health conditions affect activities	83%	16%	76%	24%
One or more hospitalizations in last year	50%	13%	45%	25%
One or more ER visits in last 6 months	48%	na	42%	17%
Reports 0–3 of 18 health conditions	52%	na	50%	100%
Reports 4–5 of 18 health conditions	23%	na	35%	0%
Reports 6 or more of 18 health conditions	25%	na	15%	0%
ADL & IADL				
Does not need help with ADLs	54%	na	24%	94%
Needs help with 1–2 ADLs	23%	na	28%	3%
Needs help with 3–5 ADLs	32%	na	48%	3%
Needs help with 0–3 IADLs	43%	na	30%	92%
Needs help with 4–6 IADLs	20%	na	17%	8%
Needs help with 7–8 IADLs	37%	na	53%	0%
Mobility				
Can walk up and down stairs	25%	na	12%	88%
Uses a wheelchair	34%	na	53%	4%
Equipment				
Uses 0–2 of 10 items	59%	na	63%	86%
Uses 3–4 of 10 items	22%	na	33%	10%
Uses 5 or more of 10 items	18%	na	4%	4%

TABLE 4.1 *(Continued)*

	Care Receivers (N = 418)	Care Givers (N = 467)	Adult Foster Homes[b] (N = 296)	NORCs[c] (N = 114)
Living arrangements				
Lives alone	10%	11%	1%	na
Lives with spouse	46%	62%	3%	na
Lives with child(ren) or other relative	37%	24%	2%	na
Lives with non-relative(s)	8%	3%	93%	na
Current housing type				
My own residence . . .	69%	na	2%	95%
The residence of a friend . . .	18%	na	1%	3%
Group home, board and care, nursing home, other	12%	na	97%	2%
Current marital status				
Married	51%	74%	16%	41%
Widowed, divorced, or separated	41%	19%	77%	47%
Never married	8%	7%	7%	11%
Race				
White	75%	71%	97%	72%
Black or African American	10%	12%	0%	0%
Asian or Pacific Islander	9%	10%	1%	28%
Other	5%	7%	1%	0%
(Hispanic origin)	7%	7%	0%	1%
Female	58%	78%	78%	62%

[a] For items included in counts of conditions, ADLs, IADLs, and equipment, see Table 3.1.
[b] For AFH project, health condition counts are 4–6 and 7 or more. IADL counts are 0–2, 3–6, & 7 or 8. Equipment counts are 0–3, 4–6, and 7 or more.
[c] For NORC project IADL counts are 0, 1-3, and 4 or more. Equipment counts are 0–2, 3–6, & 7 or more.

Care receivers were, of course, much more ill and dependent (as rated by their caregivers): Nearly two-thirds were rated to have fair or poor health; four of five had health conditions that affected their activities; and 48% had four or more chronic health conditions (Table 4.1). About half had been in the emergency room in the last 6 months or the hospital in the last 12 months. Nearly one-third needed help with three or more ADLs, and 37% needed help with seven or eight IADLS. More than a third used a wheelchair, and 40% used three or more types of adaptive equipment. More than two-thirds of the care receivers lived in their own homes, but 12% lived in a group home or nursing home. Fifty-one percent were married, but only 46% lived with their spouse.

Hawaii tried to target new caregivers (6 months or less) who were judged to be facing a long period of caregiving. The site had difficulty attracting the caregivers of these members while the members were still in the hospital, even with door-to-door handouts and invitations to in-hospital sessions offered at various times. Overall, they constituted only 8% of initial participants. The typical caregiver-to-be wasn't able to focus on the "role" of caregiver so early and was more caught up in the emotion and anxiety of the moment. Also, caregivers disliked the term "caregiver" and needed it explained to them. Ultimately, Hawaii was similar to the other sites in attracting veteran, older caregivers who were at a point where they realized that they needed help. In a similar vein, the Denver site tried to target caregivers for children with disabilities, but very few attended.

The survey of 59 non-participants found that the most common reasons for not attending were the schedule (27%), location (27%), and lack of respite (14%). The most urgent needs reported by non-participants were respite (24%) and emotional support (19%). When asked the best way to get their needs met, the most common response was "don't know" (19%), while others cited services supports, respite, and help with coping skills. The data indicate that time and location were important. Kaiser Permanente clinics are one-half hour apart and that may be too far to drive, particularly for elders in urban areas. A staff member from the Carter Institute said they usually gave workshops in towns of 20,000 to 35,000, where distance was less and easier and where there were fewer alternative ways to get this kind of information.

There were some vexing cases among non-participants. One employed daughter caring for her parents said her parents had completely isolated themselves: "They want me around 24 hours a day. They want to totally consume me." She saw her only solution to be "through my parents' death." One of the help-line nurses supported these portraits of non-participants: "I think that on a cognitive level they know the workshops would be helpful, but they just don't make it a priority. When they are in a crisis and it is a priority, they can't devote this kind of time to come to a workshop." A supervising geriatrician from the Hawaii site added this: "The caregivers most in need of support actively avoid participation." The project's practice was to refer those who signed up but did not attend to social services for follow up support. Hawaii referred many caregivers to the Alzheimer's Association, since most were caring for dementia patients. This suggests future exploration of services to these high risk families, for example, through specially designed home health caregiver support programs (Archbold & Stewart, 1996).

Participant Impact and Feedback

Participants were very satisfied with the workshops in terms of the quality of instruction, content, organization, facilities, amenities, and overall. On a four-point scale (4 = very satisfied), the percent of respondents indicating "very satisfied" ranged from 65% to 89%, with higher ratings in the later sessions of the three-to-five session series. Positive comments (see Box 4.2) focused on group discussion, support from other caregivers, recognizing positive and negative emotions, and problem-solving techniques.

The participants also judged the training workshops to be successful in increasing their preparedness and enjoyment of caregiving, and in reducing the number who often felt sad or depressed. Analyses reported in more detail in a separate paper on the project (Leutz, Capitman et al., 2002) showed that on all preparedness items, scale scores were significantly higher in the follow-up. Most change (nearly one scale point) was in the areas of finding out about and setting up services, including the health system. Least change (.24 points) was in increased enjoyment of caregiving, but enjoyment was high to start with, so didn't have as far to increase. There was an average improvement of two-thirds of a point in the nine-item preparedness scale. There was a 12-point drop in the proportion often feeling sad or depressed (from 47% to 35%).

BOX 4.2   Participant Comments

"Small groups, laughing, and ways to manage stress were helpful."

"Made me examine why negative emotions occur and what coping skills I can use."

"It was helpful to get a list of local resources. I had no idea what was out there."

"Thank you—Thank you—Thank you to Kaiser for making this program available."

Regression analyses found that there was more improvement in preparedness and reduced sadness/depression

- for caregivers who were married
- for caregivers who were employed
- when more sessions were attended
- when the caregiver was older.

Additionally, more improvement in preparedness only was found

- for caregivers whose health was good or excellent
- for caregivers who cared fewer hours
- for caregivers who helped with more IADLs
- when the caregiver was not the care receiver's spouse
- when the care receiver was a male.

Additionally, reduction in depression for the caregiver was more likely when

- the caregiver did not live with the care receiver
- the care receiver's health was not excellent
- the care receiver was less often in the emergency room
- the care receiver was Hispanic
- the care receiver was not male
- the location was not California
- the prescore was higher.

Provider Feedback

Only the Mid-Atlantic site surveyed providers about the project. Half of the 49 respondents said they seldom or never referred caregivers to internal support resources; 65% seldom or never referred to the community; 55% didn't know about community resources to support caregivers; and 35% did not feel confident they could identify family caregivers at risk of failing in their caregiving role. Three-quarters felt the health plan should provide caregiver support as a routine part of the primary health care team, and 61% said they would like to receive training about incorporating caregiver support into their practice. Their top five concerns/needs related to providing help to family caregivers were poor knowledge of services (28% of respondents), lack of time (25%), cost of support services (18%), skills to assess caregiver readiness (16%), and staff training (13%).

Systems Learning

Besides reaching out to members, the caregiver project tried to make internal systems changes, particularly in the area of enlisting providers to help identify and refer caregivers. Although project staff worked to educate providers about the project, they did not get much help in the way of referrals. This was a contrast to the relatively good support for the dementia project reported in the next chapter. The Hawaii coordinator found that gaining interest of KP providers was "the most disappointing part of the entire project":

> My challenge was to educate and encourage my co-workers on the benefits of the workshops because there was need for the "buy in." I never understood the concept of a "buy in," but it was explained to me that staff, including physicians, nurses, social workers and discharge coordinators were simply too busy to take time to explain a prevention method when the daily discharge needs were ever present. [The irony is that] the most effective method of recruitment was personal invitation from a caring staff member involved.

The Riverside coordinator learned not to expect much help from providers:

> Physician groups tend to have too much on their plate to even schedule our program in. Furthermore, they have more immediate needs for the patient and may not have needs of the caregiver as a priority. I get calls about every day from caregivers and never from providers. They don't seem to want to be bothered with having to talk about something else for the patient. They tend to be a skeptical group and want to be assured it will work. They have to believe it is a reliable support program in which the patient is not going to go back to them with "why did you send me there?" In some ways I don't blame them. . . . That's why in our caregiver program we marketed right to the member and not so much the provider. We did do prescription pad style referral slips but it is the member's responsibility to contact us. We would never expect the provider to refer someone to us directly.

The situation was much the same in Denver. During the implementation stage it was difficult to get on the calendar to meet with providers, and site leaders decided to not pursue that tactic aggressively. Rather, they decided to solicit referrals from care managers prior to each course offering and emphasized the use of flyers in displays in waiting areas.

Although physicians and care coordinators were less directly involved with the caregiver project than some of the others, project leaders found enough support to continue at two of the four sites after the demonstration officially ended in January 2000. Colorado offered caregiver training workshops quarterly through four community partners: Easter Seals of CO, the Rocky Mountain Stroke Association, the Alzheimer's Association, and the Multiple Sclerosis Society. The four partners each covered roughly a quadrant of the service area. Kaiser Permanente paid the partners' facilitators at the rate it paid health educators ($30/hour), and the information/registration line was staffed with volunteers. Advertising continued in local publications, on the Web site, and through fliers in KP facilities. In the year after the study period ended, there was a steady flow of health plan members, with 11–18 in attendance per session.

Riverside provided its own trainers and space after the study period in one of two participating medical centers. Advertising was cut back to distributing prescription pads for physicians and, about two weeks before new sessions, putting fliers in the 40 or so display holders near elevators in the hospital and clinic. In the first ten months, this yielded about ten calls a month, plus another 18 from clinical and member referrals. With the lighter demand, workshops were extended to every other week; to reduce waiting time, new members were encouraged to start at any point in the sequence. All this yielded steady attendance of about 12 caregivers per session. Additionally, a lay person continued to lead a monthly support group with an average of 12 participants. The format was a 90 minute session split between open discussion followed by a speaker—e.g. from the Alzheimer's Association, financial planning for long-term care, and the Office on Aging.

Summary

Caregiving workshops were useful for preparing caregivers for their responsibilities, but were more useful for some than for others. Those helped most in preparedness tended to be managing care rather than providing care full-time. They were married but not to the care receiver, and they were not living with the care receiver. Similarly, caregivers whose sadness/depression was reduced were working and married but not living with the care receiver. Although no statistical test was performed to explain lack of progress, it's a good guess that those who were married to and living with the care receiver achieved relatively smaller increases in preparedness and lower reductions in depression/sadness. Many others were not helped at all because they could not manage to attend. The two latter groups—those helped less or not at all—may have some characteristics in common, including factors associated with higher risks. Understanding who these caregivers were can help shape other interventions more appropriate to their needs.

These findings support the value of offering caregiving workshops, and a large managed care plan appears to be a good place to identify customers. About half of those calling the caregiver help line started the workshops; most participants finished; and many reported significant benefits. Demand was less than demonstration planners expected, but that is part of learning and not necessarily bad news. Lower demand translates to lower costs of offering the service.

The findings also support the need for additional and alternative caregiver supports, especially for full-time, resident, spousal caregivers. Additional factors related to non-completion included caring for someone who is in poor and unstable health and being in poor health oneself. One helpful array of services would be respite and transportation. These would not only allow these caregivers to attend workshops, but would also allow time off for other reasons. Another array of services would be informational and emotional support offered to caregivers through more traditional case management programs. Help in these areas may be logical extensions of caregiving workshops. For example, workshops at the Riverside site spawned caregiver support groups that continued after workshops ended. Given the clear physical and mental health risks from full-time, stressful caregiving—especially for resident spouses—strong arguments can be made for strengthening such supports through other funding sources. As mentioned earlier, there is evidence that intensive caregiver assessment and support could be beneficial in the design of home care services.

Finally, this project also holds lessons about linking with community agencies—lessons that are relevant to the previous and next chapters. The ways that the KP regions offered caregiver workshops shows yet more ways to partner with community agencies. Use of the Carter Center curriculum eased development, lent to success, and enhanced the reputations of both organizations. Locally, after surveying the community care landscape, some regions chose to offer the workshops themselves in health plan facilities, while others helped a community agency to offer and fill the workshops. The KP Denver group paid for the instructors to lead workshops offered in community agencies, and community agency staff appreciated this, since it recognized the value they believed they were providing to KP members. The difficulties gaining physicians' attention supports one of the "laws of integration" discussed in Chapter 1 ("your integration is my fragmentation") and is also a lesson for the projects discussed in Chapter 5. Fortunately, alternative ways of identifying and connecting with caregivers were found.

ADULT FOSTER CARE PILOT

The Developers and Their Goals

Given the intense national interest in more affordable and less institutionalized congregate living alternatives to nursing home care, the proposal to improve linkages with members residing in adult foster home (AFHs) in Portland was welcome. The development team, led by the manager of continuing care services and a regional nursing consultant, had conducted a preliminary search of a database that tracks admissions and discharges for hospitals, nursing facilities, and other institutions, and identified 600 members in AFHs. The interdisciplinary design team also included a social worker, an adult nurse practitioner, a physician, two primary care nurses, a pharmacist, a care coordinator, a hospital discharge coordinator, a Social HMO resource coordinator, a continuing care/home health nurse, and two researchers. The plan to include two AFH caregivers was not realized.

The team's proposal detailed the frailty of these members, the challenges tracking and serving them in primary care settings, and the risks associated with small residential programs staffed by paraprofessionals. The team proposed analysis of AFH resident medical care utilization patterns, a needs assessment using the health status survey, and concurrent development of a replicable primary care model for AFH residents that would facilitate greater participation in care decision making by residents, family members, and AFH caregivers. The needs assessment and model development were scheduled for the first 6 months, to be followed by a 6-month implementation and testing period.

Planning, Development, and Implementation

In the first phase of the project, the team met twice a month to guide development. The HSF survey and comparative analysis of utilization data were conducted using existing survey and data analysis capabilities in the Center for Health Research. Results are reported presently. The bigger planning task was to systematically learn about issues in caring for AFH members and to develop a model of care. In meetings with state officials, the team learned about the complexity and fragmentation of the external AFH regulatory system. Internally, case studies identified numerous issues, including shortcomings in primary care providers' understanding of health plan benefits relevant to AFH members; poor communication between the health plan and AFH caregivers (in part due to cultural differences that also affected caregivers' communication with residents[1]); barriers to communication and coordination between hospital, home health, and primary care; lack of a system to track transitions of AFH members (e.g., home → AFH, AFH → hospital → AFH, AFH → AFH); and end-of-life management problems.

The care management model that resulted from this investigation had three key components:

1. approaches to care coordination during transitions,
2. minimum standards of health assessment/medical evaluation, including information on the AFH care environment, and
3. inclusion of care plans in the health plan's existing on-line care management system.

Because of resource constraints, the third component was not piloted.

---

[1] A large proportion of foster care providers in Oregon are Rumanian immigrants.

Characteristics of Members Served

The Demonstration's HSF was mailed to 560 AFH resident members identified in health plan discharge records. They returned 296 surveys (53% return rate), 269 of which (91%) were from members age 65 or over. Compared to the individuals served by other projects in the demonstration, these members were extremely frail and medically complex (Table 4.1). The health of 61% was rated fair to poor compared to others of the same age, but this is a difficult to interpret since half the respondents were age 85 or over, and proxy completion was assumed to be high. Over three-quarters had health conditions that interfered with daily activities, needed help bathing, and/or needed help taking medications. More than half used wheelchairs. Not surprisingly, like the nursing home population, this was primarily a population of single, older women; and like the aged Portland population, it was overwhelmingly White.

Table 4.1 shows high rates of hospital and emergency department use, but the study team's knowledge of problems with access to routine care prompted them to look more closely at health plan utilization data. The fear was that AFH residents had relatively low clinic visit rates and correspondingly low rates of preventive care. These fears were confirmed in comparisons with other KP Northwest Medicare populations.

The first portion of Table 4.2 shows that AFH residents were higher users of hospitals but lower users of office visits compared both to KP's regular Medicare members and to the relatively older and more disabled Social HMO population. Among AFH residents, non-respondents to the HSF survey were even higher hospital users than respondents and even lower users of outpatient clinics. Not surprisingly, the second portion of the table shows that AFH resident respondents to the HSF received preventive services less often than other KPNW members who returned HSF surveys.[2] The final portion of Table 4.2 compares the utilization of the AFH survey population to the utilization of a sample of 50 AFH members who died during the year of the project. These data show that the members who died had even lower office visit rates than surviving AFH residents. There was 23% mortality in the year of the project.

In summary, these data reinforced the belief that AFH resident members had relatively low utilization of the KP primary care system, and they pointed to questions about whether AFH caregivers and family were effective participants during ambulatory visits.

---

[2] The high proportion of SA II members in the survey is due to the fact that the Social HMO population is surveyed annually, while the SA population is surveyed only on entry to SA.

TABLE 4.2   Utilization by Services by Group

	Office Visits/1000	Hospital Days/1000
1. Administrative data on office and hospital use (1998)		
General Medicare	8290	945
Social HMO	9765	1515
AFH Respondents	7955	1802
AFH Non-resp.	6858	2212

	AFH	Other KPNW Aged (90% SA II; 48% aged 80+)
2. HSF data on preventive services use		
Flu injection	69%	80%
Pneumonia injection	56%	68%
Mammogram in 2 yrs.	28%	66%
	(10% unsure)	(4% unsure)

	Office Visits	ER Visits	Hospital DC/1000
3. Administrative data on proportions with office and ER visits and hospital discharge rates			
AFH Decedents	82%	62%	1040
AFH Respondents	91%	40%	413
AFH Non-respondents	89%	45%	537

Services Provided

The pilot test of the AFH care management model was conducted in two KP clinics with the highest concentration of AFH members (129 members between the two, 58 of whom returned HSFs). Kaiser Permanente knew these 129 members were there from the quarterly census of institutionalized members that is conducted by continuing care. To see whether and how suboptimal patterns of clinic care could be changed, two nurse care managers each spent 8 hours a week implementing the case management model, concentrating first on members who returned HSFs, but ultimately attempting to contact 68 residents. They began by reviewing HSFs and medical records, visiting members' AFH caregivers, and using this information to complete seven-page care plans. Ultimately, care plans were completed for 35 members.

Systems Learning

The project director's review of how effectively 24 care plans were implemented revealed that behavior management was the most frequent problem reported by AFH caregivers, followed by falls and difficulty sleeping (resulting in requests for sleeping medication). Ten of the 24 charts showed no primary care provider or no visit to a primary care physician in the year before the intervention, and several others showed patterns of not keeping scheduled appointments. The team concluded from the chart audit that the care management overlay was too weak an intervention to affect how care was (and was not) delivered (e.g., there were examples of patients entering hospitals without the primary care physician or case manager knowing). They were not able to create an internal monitoring or tracking system that would alert the team concerning a member's residence status (this was supposed to appear on the problem list of each AFH member's medical record). In fact, what appeared in the problem list was mostly facts from the HSF and added by staff. The lack of a comprehensive knowledge base hampered care planning, and thus there was not much in the chart. The team found that it was virtually impossible to track AFH admissions, discharges, and transfers between homes. The poor results were confirmed by the quarterly tracking by continuing care.

Many of the vulnerable, frail, nursing-home-like AFH members were too weak and incapacitated to continue to use the standard model of care that is designed for a more mobile independent membership. Concerns tended to be met with a prescription pad, and too often the members, families, and AFH staff just sought prescriptions, which were handled through the number one utilization option: phone medical care. The project saw evidence of this in the case reviews. Also, for members with complex palliative care, end of life care, and daily care-in-place challenges, the options given to them by the medical office staff were not robust enough for the problems because they did not have the care-in-place background to teach viable solutions.

In regard to process, the care managers had difficulties fitting the work into neat blocks of time. Each nurse manager started off with two 4-hour blocks a week, but soon had to expand to more days. Still, the demands were too fragmented and too many to fit schedules. One care manager was never able to establish an effective and reliable system for AFH caregivers to reach her even to leave a message. Another difficulty was frequent turnover of AFH caregivers, although the owners were stable.

Care managers found that AFH caregivers often had difficulty getting members to primary care appointments. Transportation was part of the problem, but another part was managing behavior in the office. Some AFH caregivers were also found to be in stress or even in dangerous situations (e.g., one asked for medications to control behavior of a resident who had been thrown out of a prior home). This raised the question of the medical care system's responsibility for reporting fragile caregiving if it doesn't involve abuse.

In addition to the care plan review, after several months of the pilot, the team reviewed medication regimes for 26 other patients and directed a group of graduate nursing students in a sub-study of 50 decedents (deceased members). These studies revealed additional challenges with working with the AFH population in other KP systems. Chart reviews revealed a clear tendency toward managing medications by telephone, which is understandable for AFH caregivers but problematic without direct physical examination. Pharmacists reported fears of adverse interactions and inability to assess this without examination. Pharmacists also feared that language barriers with some AFH caregivers hampered their understanding of orders. State requirements that KP fax notice of all prescription and over-the-counter drug changes also created a heavy workload for the pharmacy.

The review of 50 decedent charts found that not one had a Physician's Orders for Life-Sustaining Treatment (POLST) form completed and signed by the elder and his/her primary care physician (Narizny, Perkins, et al., 1999). This form appears in the problem list in patients' medical record and indicates their preferences for treatments such as cardiopulmonary resuscitation (CPR) or antibiotic treatment. It is KP's preferred form of advanced directives and is designed to follow the individual between home and treatment facilities to clarify choices about a patient's end-of-life preferences. While the POLST was missing, 14 decedents had do-not-resuscitate (DNR) orders; seven had an advanced directives form in their records; and others had one of these three buried in a dictation or more obscure section of their chart. Over half (27) of the AFH residents were enrolled in hospice before their deaths, but 18 of these were initiated within one month prior to death (10 within a week).

The overall conclusion from these studies and efforts to strengthen case management was that the model was not sufficiently robust or intensive to demonstrate improvement in coordination of care across the continuum. As the project progressed, project team actions seemed to shift from an emphasis on improving communication between health plan and AFH caregivers to a sense of urgency about improved communication between different components of the health plan's internal system. Although the project was not able to include care plans in the health plan's online care plan system, project staff were successful in having the one-page SEEK[3] summary of these data scanned into the medical record as a "self-report"

---

[3] Screen Every Elder in Kaiser, a one-page successor to the HSF screen, containing selected HSF and other items.

document for all respondents. This summary includes the member's risk score for re-hospitalization and frailty risk score. It was available to all clinical staff in the division, not just limited to the two medical offices for this project.

Provider Feedback

Project staff conducted background interviews with 19 medical office physicians and staff about their interactions with AFH staff. The survey revealed more systems problems. Providers reported that AFH patients who made it to ambulatory care found a system that was not ready for them. Problems included lack of space and equipment, the rapid visit pace, and a general assumption that patients aren't cognitively or physically impaired. Often the family brought in the patient, but the family member did not know about day-to-day care and behavior, and it was not clear what was transmitted by the family member back to the AFH caregiver. And when health plan providers did speak to caregivers, they questioned the caregivers' understanding of medical issues. Finally, when members showed up in the clinic alone, they often couldn't provide the information or participate in making decisions. Challenges were again identified with prescriptions, which were vital because 82% needed help taking medications and 36% took more than five medications a day. The provider survey showed widespread concern with the AFH caregivers' understanding and compliance with medication regimens.

Summary

The AFH project revealed a high-risk and dependent population living in a never-never land between the community and the institution. Community residents with this level of dependency generally have a responsible family caregiver who can be relied on for transportation, communication, and continuity. Nursing home residents with such intensive and extensive needs acquire a relatively strong professional and institutional support system, including requirements (and, in KP's case, clear arrangements) for primary care physicians to come to the patient on a regular basis. The AFH project team concluded that they had uncovered a much more difficult situation than they had anticipated, in terms of both the reality of the AFH setting and the inadequacy of the health plan's capacity to provide appropriate health care.

The project's recommendations (Box 4.3) focus on the health plan's responsibilities. These were followed up with the support of the continuing care physician and additional KP funding to develop and pilot an even stronger model of care. In the pilot project, the physician group agreed to increase provider staffing, which allows KP Northwest long-term care physicians and nurse practitioners to go not only to nursing homes but also to see patients in adult foster homes in an effort to provide on-sight primary care in lieu of

BOX 4.3   Adult Foster Care Recommendations
• Develop an intensive health care delivery model. • Include a reliable tracking and monitoring system. • Get continuing care to refer earlier to hospice. • Improve pharmacy connections—evaluate in the home. • Train health plan staff re AFH population and their families. • Assess health plan costs for AFH population. • Explore legal and ethical issues regarding reporting poor care, confidentiality, and autonomy. • Coordinate with state initiatives to improve AFH care and the AFH-medical interface.

emergency department or hospital use. It is the health plan's next attempt to better meet these patients needs. Also, continuing care will contract with the calling service to phone each AFH quarterly to identify current KP residents. This calling stopped in 1999 after the federal Health Care Financing Administration dropped foster home residence as an institutional payment category under the Medicare prospective payment system to HMOs. But it is clear that the infrastructure of caring needed to be strengthened on the AFH side as well. Linkage between medical care and community care can't work unless both sides have the capability to create and maintain the ties.

LINKAGES TO NATURALLY OCCURRING RETIREMENT COMMUNITIES

The Developers and Their Goals

This project sought to connect with and better serve concentrations of frail elders residing in high-rise condominiums and co-ops in Honolulu's Waikiki neighborhood. The proposal came from a KP medical social worker in Honolulu, who believed there were many under-served elders living in these buildings, based on past social service referrals received by the social workers at her clinic.

The first goal of the project was to assess the needs of all residents of selected buildings (health plan members and non-members alike). The demonstration development team asked that the demonstration's HSF be used. The second goal—added by the development team—was to create a supportive services network in the buildings. This was a modification of the social worker's original goal, which was to perform a more traditional case management role for those residents found to need help in the needs assessment.

The "naturally occurring retirement communities" (NORCs) that these buildings seemed to contain were a more diffuse sort of congregate setting than the adult foster home. There were many more residents; most were assumed to be independent; and in the absence of organizing work like that attempted in the project, there were no formal supportive services in place through the NORC itself, even though many residents were thought to need help performing instrumental and personal activities.

The supportive services system model that KP tried to create in this project involved residents, managers, and service providers in thinking through how to identify and address needs of all residents rather than helping people one at a time in the traditional case management model. It was hoped that this would lead to approaches such as schedules for supported transportation, geographic rather than individual allocation of personal care and homemaking aides, and mutual support through volunteering. Four large buildings were chosen as targets, since it was known that they housed many health plan members. Members were by no means the majority of residents, however, and there was no intention to limit the benefits of the project to health plan members, which would have been inconsistent with the supportive services model.

Planning, Development, and Implementation

Interviews with local community agencies, the State Department of Aging, and building managers substantiated the needs of building residents, including help with chore services, transportation, and social activities. Self-denial of need and preferences for privacy were said to be barriers, however. Low income was also a problem, particularly in its effect on ability to purchase services and prescription drugs. Both public and private agencies supported KP's initiative. One agency agreed to provide educational sessions and help organize volunteer networks.

With community participation looking promising, the coordinator contacted building managers to gain their agreement for the project staff to enter the buildings, talk to residents, and distribute needs assessment surveys. Although most agreed to participate, the project staff began to encounter barriers with managers, boards of directors, and residents. These difficulties provided some lessons about how to and how not to develop a supportive services network, and also about the role an organization like KP can play.

The most prominent implementation problem was with access to the buildings. The two coops and the condo that were targeted first all had member boards that employed building managers. The project coordinator's contacts were with managers, and although two quickly agreed to participate, building policies restricted the team's movements and actions. The building boards of directors had the reputation of being careful to protect the privacy of residents, particularly from solicitors, and they lived up to those reputations. They allowed a member of the team to sit in the lobby for a weekly social time. Refreshments were offered as an incentive to talk to the KP staff and complete needs assessments, but the staff was not allowed further into the buildings. The boards also had policies of not giving outsiders a roster of residents. One board relaxed this policy and let the project mail surveys to residents with a return envelope, but the two other buildings did not. In fact, the third did not allow social hours and only allowed the forms to be left on a table in the lobby. The project coordinator was never able to meet directly with the boards to sell the project, even though she asked. In the meantime, boards made decisions about participation in the project, including rescinding any access to one building (this was after the building manager left). A fourth building that was contacted never responded to phone calls or letters.

Characteristics of Participants

Given the building access problems, it was not surprising that there were problems conducting the needs assessment. But the problems seemed to go beyond restrictions in the buildings and also related to the utility of the HSF as a tool to learn about residents' needs and gain their confidence. Of the 900 health status questionnaires distributed in the three buildings, only 128 (14%) were returned, and only 114 of these returned a signed consent form to allow their data to be used.

Based on reports from the project manager and the social work students who helped her obtain the data, it appears that the resistance to completing the form came from several quarters. One problem may have been the form itself, which asked many specific, personal questions about health and functional status and demographics. Asking for a consent form (a KP regional IRB decision) also was likely a barrier. Since no clinical relationship was existing with the residents, or promised, it is not surprising that many resisted completing it. Another problem was the method for returning the form. One building manager required that the forms be returned to his mailbox, and the return rates were lowest there. Better rates were to a locked box in the lobby, and best rates were in the building where return address envelopes were provided.

There is also reason not to trust that the data reported were representative. Project staff reported that the oldest and most disabled residents seemed most likely to try to avoid them. Staff came to believe that the most at-risk residents—e.g., those with canes and walkers—did not want themselves identified, perhaps for fear that they would be forced to leave by their families or by management. A quick look at the data in Table 4.1 tends to support this view. Compared to both the AFH residents and the care receivers for the caregiver projects, the NORC respondents were much healthier, lower users of health care services, and much more independent in functioning. None reported more than three chronic health conditions, and rates of ADL limitations (6%) and IADL limitations (8%) were lower than general population norms. But 14% were using three or more types of adaptive equipment, and 24% admitted to health conditions that affected their activity levels.

Services Provided

In addition to (and perhaps because of) the difficulties developing cooperative relationships with residents and boards, the staff was not successful in developing the hoped-for partnership arrangements with community agencies. The types of relationships established were generally of the more traditional case manager to case manager type—i.e., sharing information related to referrals and the needs of common clients. The coordinator did not bring the agencies into a supportive services model. She did not see much potential for such cooperation because of the lack of cooperation from building managers and because the needs assessments identified few clients already receiving services from these agencies. Nor did she make enough referrals to create a critical mass to make it attractive for any single agency to think about the buildings as more than collections of individual clients. Most referrals were for "meals on wheels" or to the state aging agency.

There was only limited payoff for KP or its members. The percentage of health plan members in the buildings was estimated to be 20% to 25%, but this could not be confirmed because of the low return rates. Phone calls were made to known health plan members to urge them to participate in the needs assessment. Also, forms returned by members were screened, and high-risk members were contacted to discuss help needed and possible referrals. One resident joined KP.

Despite these difficulties, there was progress towards a supportive services approach in at least one of the buildings. The coordinator developed a close contact with a private home health agency, which sent out a nurse to do a workshop there. Another "agency" that came in was the fire department, which did a well-attended (30 people) workshop on fire safety. This workshop was the residents' idea, and they also asked for sessions on nutrition and safety. The project coordinator also saw an opportunity here for bringing in the lifestyle and health education department at KP for a workshop.

The coordinator also learned that building managers, with the approval of their boards, could become referral sources for residents. At least one already did this, and also performed errands for residents and carefully screened chore workers before letting them post notices in the building. She lived in the building and also had called Elder Affairs for support for residents. Over the course of the project the coordinator spent time talking to managers about identifying needs, what community resources were available, and how to contact them. One manager put resource information in the building newsletter, and another distributed a resource information brochure. However, without explicit board recognition of the need for managers to do more in this area, this would be difficult for them to fit into their jobs.

Summary

It proved difficult for the NORC project staff to assess needs of people who did not want to be assessed, and it was even harder to develop a supportive services network in buildings that spurned outsiders. Kaiser Permanente was not the first service agency to face these barriers—Elder Affairs had tried before to get into the buildings—and it is clear that a careful approach would be needed to gain trust. In retrospect, the concept of creating a supportive services model in NORCs seems like a better fit for community agencies that specialize in supportive services than for an HMO such as KP. Still, the resistance encountered from building boards, managers, and residents was real, and would-be helpers should hear the message it may be sending. People like to be left alone, and they are suspicious of outsiders, even when outsiders say they want to help. Kernels of self-help and self-definition of needs began to sprout in at least one of the communities of elders touched by this project, but time ran out.

Finally, the lessons from the AFH and NORC "partnerships" build on some of the lessons discussed in the last chapter concerning linking with community agencies. The AFH and NORC efforts were disappointments in that new linkage relationships were achieved only partially if at all. For example, the AFH project identified clear member needs and important health plan roles, but these needs and roles were more than either the foster homes or KP itself were ready to fill with the time and resources available. More fundamental changes in care management within KP are conceivable and perhaps will soon be tested, but it's not clear where AFHs will find the resources and flexibility to link more effectively with managed care.

In the case of the NORC project, neither clear member needs nor an important HMO role were identified. This is not the first time that a big health care organizations has tried to offer or manage community services better than its local community, but such efforts are seldom successful (Capitman, Prottas, et al., 1988). The KP project found some evidence that the NORC model could work in the Waikiki condos, but KP's money might have been better and more economically spent supporting a community agency lead of a long-term community coalition.

LESSONS FROM THE PROJECTS

These three projects illustrate two broad themes about the relationships between health plans and their members. Their themes concern, first, what medical care providers need to know about their frail members' community living capabilities, social situations, and support options; and second, how providers can most effectively communicate with and connect with members about these issues. In short, what's important to know, how to know it, and how to communicate in ways that connect with members and help link them with appropriate help.

First, the projects described in the last two chapters show that a complex set of objective conditions, relationships, attitudes, and linkage opportunities and barriers affects what community and health services frail members may need and how effectively they can use those services (Box 4.4). If organized medical care systems want to be effective in understanding members' needs for social support and in connecting them to community services to address unmet need, they had better find ways to gather and use this information. Physicians were generally limited partners in this enterprise, but there was evidence of their willingness to do more, e.g., the 75% feeling that KP should routinely support caregivers through the primary health care team and the 61% who would like to incorporate caregiver support into their practice. The HMO has an opportunity to offer support, which is recognized in the KP Care Management Institute motto, "Make it easy to do the right thing."

The volume of calls to the caregiver project help line revealed a broad interest among caregivers in getting support, but certain subgroups of caregivers were much more likely than others to use and benefit from the service. On the one hand, caregivers who were employed, married (but not to the care receiver), and not living with the care receiver benefited most from the workshops. Their participation justifies the service. On the other hand, full-time spouse caregivers appeared to be the least likely to even start the workshops and were also the least likely to finish if they did start. Many revealed themselves to be too trapped in caregiving to get out, or too isolated by lack of transportation to get to the workshops, or both. Setting up a service that works for some, but not for a group that has been identified at increased risk for mortality (Schulz & Beach, 1999), shows the importance of monitoring for both successes and failures. The project's practice of following up with individuals who signed up but didn't participate is one model.

Other examples of the importance of these data jump out from the AFH project. Although AFH residents were only marginally more disabled than the care receivers in the caregivers training project (or, for that matter, than many of the members served in the projects covered in the last chapter), they posed distinctly different challenges to better linking community care and

---

BOX 4.4   Things to Know about Members, Caregivers, and Their Communities

- *Objective conditions and capabilities:* member's living arrangements, functional status (ADLs and IADLs), cognitive status, wealth.
- *Relationships:* member's caregivers, their capabilities and resilience, degree of social isolation.
- *Attitudes and preferences:* member's and caregivers' sense of independence and privacy, stage in the life cycles of disability and caregiving, readiness for outside help.
- *Linkage opportunities and barriers:* transportation, location, eligibility for community care, ability to handle procedures, forms, and information.

---

medical care. Formal AFH caregivers were primary in day-to-day care, which meant that the family caregivers who were more likely to bring members to ambulatory medical care visits often lacked important information. Conversely, telephone communications with the formal AFH caregiver about medications were very different from the face-to-face communications that were more typical with family caregivers of members living in their own residences. And without a flexible family member to drive, lack of transportation for AFH residents apparently kept medical visits from happening or required substitution of an expensive and inappropriate ambulance trip to the emergency department. Finally, the lack of regular connections of AFH residents and caregivers to primary care appeared to be a factor in the low rates of advanced directives among a population that definitely should have had them.

The NORC project revealed yet another side of the member in the community: assertive of independence, suspicious of the professional, hiding or denying the extent of disability, protected from the outside by a residential community. These attitudes and attributes were not exclusive to this project. In the last chapter there was evidence of resistance to adult day services coming from frail members who did not want to leave their homes and from caregivers who questioned whether outsiders could adequately care for their family members. Some people reported that services could be more hassle than they were worth. The residents of the NORCs also often had low incomes, which blocked access to fee-for-service help.

Now the second question: How can a medical care system best communicate with and connect with members about their community care status, needs, preferences, and opportunities for help? The projects show that communications and connections are two-way: the system tries to get information to members and also wants to get information from members. These exchanges need to be structured to occur at several levels and in multiple settings. The typical linkage project wanted to reach appropriate individuals with tailored and personalized messages, while at the same time using mass messages to reach the whole community of members because project staff knew that the personalized approaches were not enough (Box 4.5). Additionally, projects showed that the point of entry to a service was a key place for two-way information exchange, and that, after entry, providers could do many things to solidify and maintain the member's connections with services.

The caregivers project was a good example of the multi-level strategy. Project leaders trained providers to recognize and refer likely candidates, and had tailored materials ready when they did. But they knew that mass communications were needed because providers would miss many members and that many more would not even have a provider contact. Once individuals were identified as interested in the service, more tailored approaches provided specific information. Members participating in focus groups said they valued easy-to-read program brochures and information sheets on community resources or issues concerning specific conditions such as diabetes.

The point of entry into a service, or just into two-way communication, should be carefully considered for its impact on access and use. The staff consensus from several projects was that a telephone call-in line was the most open and low-risk way for members and families to make an inquiry about a service. Both the caregivers project and (as will be seen in the next chapter) the Alzheimer's projects used this approach, but somewhat differently. The caregiver call-in line was the simplest—a recorded message that gave the option of getting a mailing about workshops or a call-back from a professional. The

---

BOX 4.5   Communication and Connection Strategies

- *Mass communication:* flyers, newsletter articles, posters, additions to mailings, health fairs, public service announcements, websites
- *Information from/about members:* database searches, health status surveys, focus groups
- *Tailored communication:* community resource sheets, information sheets on health conditions, program brochures, culturally appropriate materials
- *Personalized communication:* provider discussions and referrals, follow-up systems, targeted outreach (e.g., in hospitals)
- *Service entry connections:* telephone help line, single point of contact, no waiting admission, options for times and places, free or cheap help
- *Service content and process connections:* information (e.g., caregiver workshops, cooperative health care clinics), care consultation and coordination, emotional and social support (e.g., self-help groups, volunteers, counseling), removal of barriers (e.g., respite, transportation, financial subsidies), direct help (personal care, homemaker, adult day services), community organizing (e.g., supportive services)

responder to a phone call to the Alzheimer's single point of contact was a professional—either answering the phone directly or calling back from a recording. Kaiser Permanente providers were also urged to call the Alzheimer's project line for information about the project and related community resource issues. In both cases, access for the member was easy and direct to a source that could help with the specific interest, and it yielded a timely and direct response from the program. After the initial contact indicated interest, things that made it easier to actually use services included free or low-fee services, options for time and place, and not making people wait a long time to start (e.g., the caregivers' workshops being open to new members at any point in the sequence).

Other ways to reach out to the broader community are through database searches and surveys. The AFH project's combination of mailing a health screening survey to AFH residents who had been identified in a database search quickly gathered detailed information on half the target population. The data on the population and the individuals served as a good opener for discussions with AFH providers and individual members. Once in the AFH, it was easier to reach additional members who did not return the survey. In contrast, the HSF did not work well as an entry strategy in the NORC project. Would-be participants were not ready to provide personal information to a stranger offering unspecified help.

Finally, the content and process of the service itself was an important factor in making the connection with members. The projects showed that one size did not fit all, even when a need (e.g., caregiver support) was the same. Workshops were helpful to many caregivers, but more could have enrolled if transportation and respite care barriers had been removed. Others who reached the call-in line may have done fine with a piece of tailored communication, but some needed more intensive consultation and connection to direct services. Having the added dimension of caregiver support groups was another way to connect, as KP already knows from its positive experience with group clinic visits for patients with chronic conditions in common (Beck, Scott, et al., 1997).

In conclusion, success with community care linkage depends in large part on how a health plan reaches out to frail members about community care, learns about their needs and their lives, facilitates their entry and use, and offers options that fit varied situations and preferences. Health plan providers need to remember that for members, asking for help, processing information, and using services all take time and effort, and even a psychological toll. Moreover, the available services are seldom a perfect fit and are sometimes a poor fit. Paradoxically, individuals who are most in need of help may have the most difficulty locating and using help. Sometimes elders and families make do without help even though they want help, and sometimes they use ill fitting services out of necessity. A linkage program that can effectively provide members with information, learn more about member needs and preferences, make the entry process smoother, and facilitate better and more frequent fits with services is on its way to doing its job.

REFERENCES

Archbold, P. G., & Stewart, B. J. (1996). The nature of the caregiving role and nursing interventions for caregiving families. *Advances in gerontological nursing* (pp. 133–156). New York: Springer.

Archbold, P. G., Stewart, B. J., et al. (1992). The clinical assessment of mutuality and preparedness in family caregivers to frail older people. In S. G. Funk, E. M. Tornquist, M. T. Champagne, & L. A. Copp (Eds.), *Key aspects of elder care* (pp. 328–339). New York: Springer.

Arno, P. S., Levine, C., et al. (1999). The economic value of informal caregiving. *Health Affairs, 18*(2), 182–188.

Bech, A., Scott, J., et al. (1999). A randomized trial of group outpatient visits for chronically ill older HMO members: The cooperative health care clinic. *Journal of the American Geriatrics Society, 45*(5), 543–549.

Callahan, J., & Lansbery, S. (1997). Can we tap the power of NORCs? *Perspectives on Aging,* January–March, 13–20.

Capitman, J. A., Prottas, J., et al. (1988). A descriptive framework for new hospital roles in geriatric care. *Health Care Financing Review,* (Suppl.), 17–26.

Doty, P., Jackson, E., et al. (1998). The impact of female caregivers' employment status on patterns of formal and informal eldercare. *The Gerontologist, 38*(3), 331–341.

Emanuel, E. J., Fairclough, D. L., et al. (2000). Understanding economic and other burdens of terminal illness: The experience of patients and their caregivers. *Annals of Internal Medicine, 132*(6), 451–459.

Haigler, D. H., Mims, K. B., et al. (1998). *Caring for you, caring for me.* Athens, GA: University of Georgia Press.

Leutz, W., Capitman, J., et al. (2002). Caregiver education and support: Results of a multi-site pilot in an HMO. *Home Health Services Quarterly, 21*(4).

Narizny, J., Perkins, M., et al. (1999). *Acute and non-acute service utilization by frail elderly adult foster home residents: A study of Kaiser Permanente members.* Portland, OR: Kaiser Permanente Center for Health Research and Oregon Health Sciences University.

Schulz, R., & Beach, S. R. (1999). Caregiving as a risk factor for mortality. *Journal of the American Medical Association, 282*(23), 2215–2219.

5

Looking Inward: Making Change in Complex Organizations

Walter Leutz, Janet Bath, Linda Johns, Debra Taylor, Susan Kolibaba, Ingrid Venohr, and Warren Wong

B y this point it's becoming clearer that the bigger challenges in realiz-
ing the vision of Manifesto 2005 may lie not with the health plan's
connecting with community care agencies or members but rather with
changing the health plan itself. Kaiser Permanente is a medical services and
insuring organization, and the Manifesto asks its managers and clinicians to
expand their thinking and their responsibilities to include members' community care service needs. These are people and departments that already
have complex and over-booked jobs. How could they add this component
to practice? Who should lead the effort? Will the costs be prohibitive?
What do the linkage and coordination models need to achieve to get attention and support?

The demonstration sites attempted to get three sectors of the health plan
more involved with community care service thinking: top managers and policy makers, physicians, and what might be broadly called continuing care
staff. Of these, continuing care (including social work, senior services, home
health, geriatrics) included the staff that already came closest to having
responsibility for handling frail members' needs beyond acute and skilled
services. Kaiser Permanente's Eldercare Sourcebook repeatedly references
the importance of working with informal caregivers and linking with community care services. The problem is that proposing to link with caregivers
and community care services is one thing; the demonstration sites show that
having systems and resources to do it is another.

This chapter provides case examples of how to make change within the HMO setting. Following the model of previous chapters, first the four demonstration projects will be reviewed, and then general lessons will be synthesized. The four projects relied heavily on within-KP changes for their success.

The first project was a multi-site project for post-diagnosis dementia care. One reason cited in proposals for the importance of this initiative was the perception that health plan physicians, including neurologists, were often reluctant to make a diagnosis of dementia because they felt they had so little to offer members and families after giving them such devastating news. This finding was disturbing but apparently not unique to KP (Brown, Mutran, et al., 1998; Fortinsky, 1998). The project was designed to create a system of post-diagnostic care which linked persons with dementia and their caregivers to community resources and, in the process, to encourage and facilitate earlier diagnoses.

The second and third projects tested modest but important expansions of KP home care coverage into personal care and social support services. They expanded eligibility criteria to include the inability to perform instrumental and personal care tasks—which was not enough to qualify an individual for help under traditional skilled care criteria. These projects were exceptions to the demonstration's general policy of not supporting proposals for new service benefits, but they were judged to be important, given studies questioning HMOs' provision of home health compared to fee-for-service practices, as well as the Medicare home health cut-back provisions of the 1997 Balanced Budget Act, which had just been passed as the demonstration began.

The San Diego site expanded home health by creating "community health workers" as extensions of the continuing care team. The Hawaii site focused on members who faced what were likely to be temporary declines in functioning, particularly after surgery or an otherwise debilitating hospitalization. Both projects targeted members who had combinations of functional dependencies and weak social support that made clinicians wary of sending members home. The key challenges in such service extensions were to define a set of patients, services, and exit criteria that did not create high, long-term costs.

The fourth project explored yet another border of traditional health care coverage—"assistive technology," including durable medical equipment and supplies. There has been a tremendous explosion in AT, but most of it is not covered by health insurance. There is a saying in the field that "Medicare stops at the bathroom door," and other rooms and functions could be easily added. Yet the project director, a social worker who was the service coordination director in the Social HMO, had seen how that program's expanded coverage and management of AT could help optimize functional independence and safety of "at-risk" members (Leutz, Capitman et al., 2001). The question posed in this demonstration site was whether increased exposure to AT and improved linkage through KP provider referrals (but without coverage) would also increase access.

DEMENTIA CARE LINKAGES

The Developers and Their Goals

The need for better care for patients with Alzheimer's Disease and related dementias was a natural for the community care demonstration, and six sites sent letters of intent in this area. Site leaders were primarily nurses and social workers from departments of geriatrics and long-term care, outpatient social workers, senior programs, continuity of care, and continuing care/senior services. The LTC Committee asked them to work together, and their common proposal was led by a researcher from the Senior Programs Department of the Denver site, with several administrative and clinical consultants. The group also proposed to partner with the Alzheimer's Association (AA) to develop and test a post-diagnosis protocol for dementia care. The AA, led by its Los Angeles chapter but including the national office, was a willing and expert partner.

Planning, Development, and Implementation

Staff from all KP sites met in Los Angeles three times during the planning and development phases to discuss current dementia care issues in their regions, to review AA materials on community care for dementia patients, and to discuss how best to connect with local chapter services. The team also met biweekly by phone for the first year and monthly thereafter.

A key cross-site planning activity was to conduct 17 focus groups with 145 family caregivers of members with dementia. Participants asked for better information about the direction of the disease, how to navigate as a caregiver, and how and where to find both emotional and caregiving support (Box 5.1). They reported that health plan physicians could do a better job making earlier diagnoses and providing information, and that there could be better coordination of care from multiple health plan providers. Problems described by caregivers included inability to reach the primary care physician, difficulty renewing prescriptions, difficulty obtaining referrals to resources within and outside the health plan, and poor follow-up care once diagnosis was made. A long list of non-medical supports was said to be hard to find, including respite care, financial and legal advice, transportation, and socialization.

BOX 5.1   Experiences of Dementia Caregivers Prior to Dementia Project (from Denver focus groups)

"We got absolutely nothing at the time he was diagnosed."

"Doctors care but don't really have the time."

"I need to know what's the right thing to do. Do I force her to go to the doctor or take her medications? How do I know what I should do?"

"The doctor just didn't explain. She said she had Alzheimer's, that her brain was shrinking, and did I have any questions. She didn't even talk to my grandmother."

"I need medical people not to underestimate the task of the caregiver. Me getting up ten times a night is just another subject to you, but for me it's life and death."

"Sharon (the project case manager) has been a very good go-between to get the doctors to do what I need to help me do my job better."

The result of the planning and development work was a project manual detailing components of a Model of Dementia Care (Figure 5.1 and Box 5.2), which identifies member needs, details a KP system of care to better understand and address needs, and shows how to link members to community services for social support. The manual includes a series of supporting materials, including a Provider Education Manual, a Community Resource Manual, an Alzheimer's booklet for members, dementia management guidelines, survey measures to assess satisfaction of members and health plan provider staff, two educational booklets for members, focus group questions, an intake flow chart and activity tracker, and sample caregiving workshop flyers.

Parallel with the national protocol development, each site worked with its local AA chapter to develop the specifics of implementation in its region. All local chapters were eager to participate, and all sites fully implemented the model.

Besides developing the community connections, a key development activity was training provider and care management staff in the model and about issues that had been identified in the focus groups and other background work. For example, the Colorado site held a region-wide video conference with internal medicine physicians, addressing diagnosis, treatment options, community partnerships, and the single point of contact. They also gave an overview of the project to neurology staff and physicians. A resource binder for managing dementia was shared with all senior care coordinators, and the manual's booklet ("They tell me I have Alzheimer's. Now what?") was adapted and distributed to multiple staff classifications. The Southern California

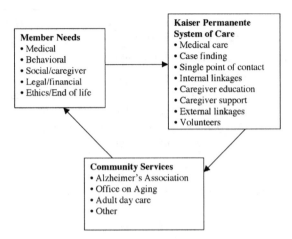

FIGURE 5.1   Model of dementia care.

site kicked off the project at medical grand rounds, attended by over 100 physicians, nurse practitioners, social workers, and nurses. The topic "update on the treatment of Alzheimer's and related dementias" was presented by a well-known physician, followed by a presentation of the project and the single point of contact and community resources. Sacramento staff held in-services at physicians' "clinic modules" (15–20 minutes) and got asked back to some departments' educational meetings (45–60 minutes). The San Francisco site translated materials into Chinese and Spanish.

Characteristics of Members Served

The members who participated in the dementia care project (as reported by their caregivers in Table 5.1) were somewhat better off in terms of several key health and functional status indicators than participants in other demonstration projects, including two of those covered in this chapter. Only 20% of the caregivers rated the health of the person they cared for as "fair" or "poor," and the proportion using five or more prescription drugs use was also reported to be low. The exception was their high rates of cognitive impairment: 50% had severe memory problems and 83% needed help taking medications. (There were several similarities to the participants in the Community Health Workers project, which we will see shortly was targeted at members with dementia.) The proportion needing help with three or more ADLs (36%) was highest among the projects in this chapter, but not as high as the 50% plus in the referral and adult day services projects. The 64%

**BOX 5.2 Key Recommendations for Implementing
the Dementia Model**

Case finding: Target both existing and newly diagnosed members. Educate physicians and staff through workshops, in-services, brochures, and web sites. Educate members through newsletter articles, mailings, brochures, and so forth. Screen HSF for report of severe memory problems.

Single point of contact: Establish a voice mail or live answer number. Follow up to assess needs, provide information, and refer to internal or community services.

Internal linkages: Establish relationships with primary care, health education, home health, nursing home team, neurology, and the emergency department.

Education: Teach health plan providers about Alzheimer's disease, member needs (from focus groups), single point of contact, care manager support, and linkages with community agencies. Teach caregivers through literature, courses, support groups, one-on-one, and referrals to Alzheimer's Association, Office on Aging, and other agencies.

Intake: Collect basic data for patients and caregivers upon initial contact, including a consent for information sharing with the AA. With consent, mail AA educational materials to members in need, and fax their names to the AA to initiate contact rather than waiting for the member to call.

AA care plan for referred members/families: AAs develop care plans for all referred members and share these plans with the health plan.

Implementation monitoring: Track outcome measures, including movement toward implementing the Model.

---

needing help with seven or eight IADLs shows the close supervision that caregivers had to provide these members. That the limitations were generally not in physical function, however, is seen in the relatively low rates of use of adaptive equipment (only 20% using three or more items). Dementia project participants were least likely to be living alone and most likely to be living in a congregate setting.

A problem behavior supplement to the HSF found that in the last five days before completing the form, more than two-thirds had become irritated/angry, restless/agitated, and repeated questions/stories. Other occurrences in the same period included bowel/bladder accidents (43%), keeping caregiver up at night (35%), and swearing (24%). Few were receiving community agency services at intake, including homemaker/aide (8%), social worker (6%), adult day services (5%), transportation (4%), visiting nurse (4%), and home delivered meals (3%).

TABLE 5.1 Participant Characteristics[a]

	Dementia Care (N = 594)	Community Health Workers[b] (N = 53)	Temporary Decline (N = 50)	Assistive Technology (N = 29)
Health condition				
Self-rated health fair or poor	20%	47%	52%	73%
Takes 5 or more prescription drugs	30%	37%	62%	48%
Severe memory problems	50%	54%	6%	3%
Health conditions affect activities	26%	na	80%	83%
One or more hospitalizations in last year	31%	29%	92%	24%
One or more ER visits in last 6 months	39%	38%	82%	41%
Reports 0–3 of 18 health conditions	57%	49%	40%	82%
Reports 4–5 of 18 health conditions	33%	36%	50%	18%
Reports 6 or more of 18 health conditions	10%	15%	10%	0%
ADL & IADL				
Does not need help with ADLs	41%	59%	18%	61%
Needs help with 1–2 ADLs	23%	17%	48%	21%
Needs help with 3–5 ADLs	36%	24%	34%	18%
Needs help with 0–3 IADLs	20%	40%	18%	64%
Needs help with 4–6 IADLs	16%	32%	58%	25%
Needs help with 7–8 IADLs	64%	28%	24%	11%
Mobility				
Can walk up and down stairs	na	na	14%	45%
Uses a wheelchair	19%	19%	24%	10%
Equipment				
Uses 0–2 of 10 items	80%	82%	42%	64%
Uses 3–4 of 10 items	14%	18%	42%	32%
Uses 5 or more of 10 items	6%	0%	16%	4%

TABLE 5.1 *(Continued)*

	Dementia Care (N = 594)	Community Health Workers[b] (N = 53)	Temporary Decline (N = 50)	Assistive Technology (N = 29)
Living arrangements				
Lives alone	22%	39%	55%	21%
Lives with spouse	45%	37%	15%	52%
Lives with child(ren) or other relative	23%	20%	26%	24%
Lives with non-relative(s)	11%	4%	4%	3%
Current housing type				
My own residence . . .	74%	76%	96%	90%
The residence of a friend	12%	15%	2%	0%
Group home, board and care, nursing home, other	14%	8%	2%	9%
Current marital status				
Married	51%	47%	16%	69%
Widowed, divorced, or separated	47%	49%	64%	30%
Never married	2%	4%	20%	0%
Race				
White	84%	82%	52%	10%
Black or African American	4%	6%	0%	0%
Asian or Pacific Islander	9%	4%	32%	0%
Other	3%	8%	16%	0%
(Hispanic origin)	na	13%	2%	0%
Female	62%	61%	60%	59%

[a] For items included in counts of conditions, ADLs, IADLs, and equipment, see Table 3.1
[b] Categories for Health conditions are 4–6 and 7 or more; IADLs are 0–2, 3–6, & 7–8; Equipment are 0–3 & 4–6, & 7 or more.

Services Provided

One year into the project, surveys measured activities and satisfaction of caregivers, providers, and community agency staff. Caregivers reported substantial increases over baseline in the use of community support services, including the Alzheimer's Association connection, support groups, and adult day services, and their satisfaction rates were high (Table 5.2). More than a quarter had used nursing homes or other supported congregate living. Compared to the utilization rates reported above, the table also shows significant numbers of caregivers using the new health plan support services, including the nurse advice line, the single point of contact, caregiver support, and Alzheimer's education. Primary care physicians were the most frequently used medical service. The proportions satisfied with health plan services ranged from 72% to 90%.

Participant Impact and Feedback

In addition to questions about these specific services, the survey measured overall satisfaction and found it to be high regarding information given about the diagnosis (76%), information about community services (85%), and sensitivity/respect shown the patient (80%). There was a diagnosis of memory loss or dementia by a health plan physician for 76% of the patients, and 64% received information from physicians about dementia-related services outside the health plan.

Provider Feedback

Of the 132 providers surveyed (61 physicians, 20 nurse practitioners/physicians assistants, 51 nurses, social workers and case managers), 85% reported that dementia services had improved from one year earlier, and 86% reported that KP gave them adequate support in their work with patients and caregivers. At least one site (Colorado) reported that the vast majority of families came from direct referrals from providers rather than the dementia call-in line.

Non-provider staff emphasized the importance to members and families of having a definite diagnosis. Until a diagnosis had been made, families did not move forward in planning for and anticipating the many challenges they faced. These staff also felt physicians could benefit from increased education about the importance of providing a diagnosis, at least acknowledging the emotional and behavioral aspects of dementia, and making appropriate referrals.

Community agencies also reported satisfaction with the health plan's dementia care initiatives, particularly regarding increases in referrals and helpfulness of the single point of contact. Before the project they didn't know who to call when they had a KP patient. Reasons they said they might

TABLE 5.2 Caregivers' Use of and Satisfaction with Community Resources (after implementation of Dementia Project) (*N* = 594)

Service	% Used	% Satisfied*
Alzheimer's Association	30	95
Support groups	20	91
Board & Care/Assisted Living	16	73
Adult Day Services	15	87
Personal Care/Chore	14	84
Educational programs	13	100
Nursing Homes	12	78
Respite Care	9	100
Caregivers' Use of and Satisfaction with Kaiser Services		
Primary Care Physician	68	84
Nurse Advice Line	33	86
Emergency Department	32	76
Single Point of Contact	29	87
Caregiver Support Program	25	90
Hospital	25	84
Psychiatry	21	82
Neurology	19	72
Alzheimer Education Program	18	86

* Either "satisfied" or "very satisfied" on a 4-point scale.

want to call included referring patients who they thought might need intensive care management (e.g., for family education, assistance connecting with community resources, home safety assessment, nursing home placement), a dementia medical workup and/or mental status testing, or just assistance navigating the KP system. During the project, the contact person assured members and AA professional staff that they would be talking to a health plan staff member who knew dementia and who would respond. Also, the AA expressed appreciation to those physicians who sent a note showing that they knew about and valued their involvement with a family. The AA was ready to provide education about non-medical aspects of dementia to physicians in sessions as short as 15 minutes.

However, concerns were raised by some local AAs. Some were frustrated at doing so much to assist KP members in ways that benefit the health plan as an organization, but without commensurate recognition and support from the health plan. For example, some staff felt that the health plan could have been more flexible in using its own services to extend more help to members—e.g., home health to do in-home assessment and crisis intervention. The concerns about lack of direct support were not universal, since at one

local AA, KP made a substantial annual financial contribution; and KP managers and staff participated on the AA board, research committee, public policy committee, and patient and caregiver education and support committee.
Overall, the chapters felt strongly that the collaboration was a good thing
because the AA's mission is to serve persons with dementia and their caregivers within their communities. The Denver chapter of AA was so pleased
with the collaboration that they subsequently offered the direct referral
model to other managed care organizations throughout the state.

Systems Learning

Each site linked with existing community resources that had previously been
underused, if used at all, and sites also found new ways to connect members
with services. The Sacramento site, for example, had a care management goal
of "following" not "managing" patients (i.e., don't be calling them all the
time), so they developed a quarterly newsletter to communicate. Once a
referral was made the family went on the mailing list. Agencies started calling in with information for the newsletter on how to do referrals and also
with events. Sites found and used community resources for in-services, caregiver training, home visits, and dementia evaluations (Box 5.3). Kaiser
Permanente participation in community agency events and committees was
noted and appreciated by community care agencies, and it also reinforced the
consciousness of health plan staff members about the supports available to
members and families.

The dementia project provided important lessons about making internal
connections. One was that each local situation had opportunities that could
be used to ease project implementation. In one site this involved using an

---

BOX 5.3   Community Connections in Dementia Projects
• Newsletter to communicate with families and KP and community providers about project services and other resources.
• In-services and literature from Alzheimer's Association for KP nursing and social work staff.
• Caregiver training classes (with free respite care) from a community provider.
• Link with county geriatric network for crisis home visits and university research center for enhanced dementia evaluations.
• Kaiser Permanente participation in community agency fund raisers (e.g., KP team in AA Memory Walk), committees, speakers bureaus, and boards.[1]

---

[1] Of course, KP members participate in these events, too. Since KP has substantial market
share in many of its west coast communities, members are supporting themselves through
these events.

existing team for the single point of contact, and in another it meant setting up a new team that continued after the official end of the demonstration (Box 5.4). In one site, subspecialists connected well to the project, while in at least one other, they did not.

The dementia project's clinical and linkage messages seemed to resonate with health plan clinicians and care management staff more readily than did some of the other projects. Perhaps this was due to effective work by project leaders, but more likely it was due to the more discrete nature of dementia compared to broad and varied natures of physical disabilities. It also may be that physicians are central to the diagnosis of dementias and are looked to for treatment options, which the project gave them.

But even with a discrete condition and a clear option for post-diagnosis care, the "sale" to physicians was not immediate. A Hawaii physician put it this way: "There are so many new programs that come along that it takes a while for programs to be 'incorporated.'" An administrator on the cross-site planning team had a similar insight: "Our inter-regional group came to an 'aha' that it can take up to a good two years to really establish a referral pattern from primary care. Providers are a little slow in figuring out what a program can do for them as they have so many competing issues to face." A Sacramento site leader had a little more mixed view, but still, in the end, positive:

BOX 5.4   Internal Connections in Dementia Projects

- Hawaii used the existing Referral Center for the single point of contact. Staff reported that the community linkages eased their burden with repeat phone calls.
- San Francisco set up a coordinating model of a core team of nurses and social workers for the primary care modules and community care program. This group identified and referred patients, distributed project materials, and worked directly with families of patients with dementia. Working with an advisory board, they standardized dementia diagnostic work-up criteria throughout the city.
- Subspecialists in San Francisco preferred to refer patients directly to the dementia project rather than back to the primary care physician. In response, staff developed and distributed a sub-specialty binder for neurologists, psychiatrists, and case managers in psychiatry, nephrology, and oncology.
- Sacramento tracked contacts with patients and caregivers using the hospital's existing "conferencing" message database. These notes were printed and placed in the patient's chart, including a copy to the outpatient medical record. All participants' charts had this message: "Dementia: for non-medical dementia issues, please call the A/D Program at [phone number] for assistance."

It took time for providers to understand the project was not offering "case management" or "clinic" services. Community agencies grasped it much more quickly. The project continued to get family feedback about incomplete diagnosis and inadequate communication with Kaiser providers. We did not make much impact on their practice, except in respect to utilizing our services.

Summary

The dementia project showed that small investments by a health plan can yield big returns for members. The project created good will among members and families, leveraged additional community benefits/resources for health plan members, and strengthened the health plan's internal cohesion in diagnosing dementia and connecting those diagnosed with support services. Reciprocal support relationships were established between continuing care and the project team. It really helped to have dementia experts available and to give them high visibility. All five dementia sites continued to follow the dementia protocol past the end of the demonstration.

COMMUNITY HEALTH WORKERS

The Developers and Their Goals

This project sought to make paraprofessional community health workers (CHWs) a part of the health care team with the goal of providing extra home care support to elders with dementia and to their caregivers. The proposal asked for funds to hire experienced paraprofessionals from local communities and to have them care for members whose conditions did not necessarily meet skilled home health criteria.

The proposal was developed by the manager of continuing care services, with assistance from a team that included a geriatrician, social work care coordinators, a nurse placement coordinator, quality assurance, hospital administration, and government and community affairs. Once the project made it into the proposal stage, developers asked if the CHW project could be integrated administratively and clinically with the dementia and volunteer projects, which had also been approved in the San Diego region. This proposal for a three-level improvement in services to members with dementia was approved by the LTC Committee.

Planning, Development, and Implementation

In the first 6 months of the project, five caregiver focus groups were held, a project coordinator was hired, CHWs were hired and trained, evaluation and operational protocols were developed, and home visits started. A steering committee from different departments met weekly throughout the development and early operational period. Internally, there were significant in-kind contributions from continuing care, administration, quality resource management, organizational effectiveness, volunteer services, and public affairs. Project staff found that provider "buy in" was fostered by involving them in the planning process and project development/implementation.

The San Diego project managed the CHW project in conjunction with the volunteer and dementia projects. Each sub-project had its own organization and process, but the joint project had monthly "integrated IRCOA meetings" with a dozen people meeting for about one-and-a-half hours. Agenda items included budget, Institutional Review Board process, job descriptions, personnel policies, recruiting and hiring, community agency meetings, workplans/reports, evaluation, and training.

The planning group's design for the roles of CHWs was based on the focus group findings and the National Community Health Advisory Study of core roles of community health advisors in health care teams. The shorthand term used by the team was to be "provider extenders" and to serve as "eyes and ears" in the home and community, but there was definitely a hands-on component in the community (Box 5.5). The site recruited, hired, and trained CHWs, who were ethnic minorities affiliated with local neighborhood health programs. The pilot project utilized four CHWs for 20 hours per week each.

Senior Services Care Coordinators recruited participants among members 65 and over and diagnosed with dementia. They also had to be "frail"—i.e., to have confusion or memory impairment, significant impairment in ADLs or medication management, and a limited support system, resulting in an inability to meet their own health and social needs. Half of the patients enrolled in the first three months, establishing base caseloads ranging from 7 to 16 per CHW. The site collected health status questionnaire data on

---

BOX 5.5   Community Health Worker Roles

- Health education and information
- Help with basic needs (e.g., nutrition, medication management)
- Access to health plan services (e.g., scheduling, referrals, follow-up)
- Help with outside services (e.g. phone, utilities, referral and follow-up to community)
- Liaison between caregivers and care coordinator re information and forms
- Advocacy re legal and other areas
- Support, encouragement, reassurance, reaffirmation, active listening, helping through the unfamiliar
- Other (e.g., documentation, scheduling)

members served in coordination with prior Senior Advantage HSF administration. Ongoing process, daily activity logs, progress notes, and telephone satisfaction surveys were conducted, and pre/post caregiver burden was assessed.

Characteristics of Members Served

A total of 55 dementia patients and their caregivers were served over the course of the project's operating year. Their mean age was 82. The HSF results from the 53 participants who returned forms (Table 5.1) show that 61% were female and that half had severe memory problems, as rated by their caregivers. There were some interesting differences between the San Diego participants and the sites in the dementia care projects overall. The CHW participants were more likely to be reported in fair or poor health or to be taking five or more prescription drugs, but they were less dependent in ADLs and IADLs. Perhaps the connection of the CHW with the continuing care department fostered a focus on more medically needy individuals.

Modal living and family arrangements for care receivers were residence in their own home or apartment (84%), being married (54%), and living with the spouse (39%). Forty-three percent were widowed, divorced or separated, and 37% were living alone. Substantial minorities lived with children or other relatives (in their home or the home of the care receiver), and a small group (5%) lived in congregate quarters. These patterns suggest some of the vulnerability and instability that were reported by staff as reasons for targeting these members for extra social support.

Services Provided

The 55 members and their families received a total of 816 home visits by the CHWs—nearly 70 visits a month on average. The average visit time was one hour. CHWs could do things that were important but not appropriate for Care Coordinators. Service logs showed CHWs providing referrals to community agencies, helping to fill out forms, setting up and following up on health plan appointments, picking up medication refills, and otherwise helping to implement care plans that were set up by health plan social workers. Community linkages that were facilitated through CHWs included meals on wheels, senior centers, Retired Senior Volunteer Program (RSVP), the Alzheimer's Association, long-term care facilities, and medical equipment.

The CHWs believed that demented elders would not have made these linkages at all without their help. Completing forms was a key link to many basic services, including utilities, landlords, etc. The CHWs also helped members complete durable medical power-of-attorney forms. CHWs also helped patients and caregivers navigate an often complex managed care system, including making or checking on health appointments with continuing care, primary care, member services, and health appraisal. CHWs reported that "number punching" through telephone triage trees was frustrating to patients and caregivers.

These CHW roles were complements to those of volunteers, who in this project were more focused on providing transportation, respite, and caregiver support. CHWs found volunteer transportation services essential, since sometimes they themselves faced transportation barriers. The combination of low wages, high costs of car maintenance, and increases in insurance rates posed recurrent challenges to the CHWs.

A 55-person comparison group was established from east and west portions of the county. Average age there was 80, and 60% were female. Thirty-seven patients (67%) had caregivers. There are utilization data for comparison and intervention groups, with no significant differences in anything but hospital, where there was a significantly lower rate for the CHW group.

Provider Feedback

Kaiser Permanente providers' feedback about CHWs was positive, so long as there was sufficient training, orientation, and supervision. The "eyes and ears" role of relating information to and from the community, as well as the access facilitator role, were valuable for care coordinators, physicians, and community agencies alike (Boxes 5.6 and 5.7). CHWs proved able to help with compliance monitoring for items such as medications. They were trained to ask if the patient was following orders, to provide encouragement, and to clarify. The team found that CHWs needed some guidelines about how far they could go. But the support they could give was clearly different from what a volunteer gave because it was support around the care plan.

BOX 5.6   Kaiser Permanente Provider Views of CHWs

A health plan physician: The CHW helped my patient to keep follow-up appointments, remember medication changes, and with placement in an assisted living facility. Prior to CHW services, communicated changes, tests, and referrals were not being followed by my patient. This was very helpful to me. I think it would be helpful if Kaiser hired CHWs as our social workers are taxed. For the frail elder this service can help prevent deterioration.

A KP Care Coordinator: The CHWs helped us in a number of ways—being the "eyes and ears" for our patient in the community, having someone to follow up with our patients on the care plan, and having bilingual CHWs to assist Spanish speaking patients. It was uplifting to see their enthusiasm for the job and to watch how each CHW developed her own job interests and expertise.

BOX 5.7   Community Agency Feedback on CHWs

We are a relatively new agency and the exposure that CHWs provide is always welcome. CHWs provide alternatives and resources to the frail elder and their caregiver.

There is a great need for community liaisons who can support and add to the social worker's role. With increasing demographics, our elderly and caregivers need special assistance in learning about aging issues and options for care. To have CHWs who can advocate for them and guide them through confusing care situations and be a friend is *very* beneficial and important. CHWs assist our role as a community partner.

Kaiser can be a complex system and patients need assistance in negotiating it. CHWs can help community agencies by providing additional information about Kaiser services.

The CHWs also provided basic health information to patients and caregivers, and they were trained to refer to others for more depth. Caregivers wanted information about stages of dementia, managing behavior, and caregiver self-care. Care coordinators developed scripts for CHWs to give these basics in Spanish and English.

The CHWs required ongoing supervision and training from providers, and this was organized in several ways. The CHWs received training from licensed social work care coordinators in weekly meetings that covered team building, case review, case finding, and administration. Clinical topics included maintaining boundaries and stress care techniques. Supervision was more effective when supervisors had a background that reflected the CHWs' job responsibilities. For example, if CHWs were providing support services, they needed a clinical supervisor; if their job was more medically related they did better with a nurse supervisor. CHWs also attended monthly seminars and workshops in the community related to dementia and caregiving. These offered unusually extensive training and close supervision for paraprofessional home care workers.

Care coordinators reported that solid up-front training and orientation were essential, including reading, job shadowing, documentation, and visiting community agencies. CHWs asked for a more structured training curriculum that included educational tools, patient/caregiver handouts, and educational scripts to help them perform their duties. Also recommended were attending refresher courses, volunteer training, and support groups.

Training in documentation topics needed more work than initially envisioned, including better charting of what they did and what impacts were. Kaiser Permanente professional staff relied on the CHWs to collect data on their own activities and on caregiver burden and satisfaction. Sometime into the project they realized they hadn't given adequate training to the CHWs concerning importance of each of the evaluation components and how they fit together.

The care coordinators believed that the help that the CHWs provided more than made up for the additional time in supervision, and the numbers support this belief. During the course of the project, care coordinators took on 32% more cases than the year before the program.

Summary

The CHW project worked in conjunction with the San Diego region's dementia and volunteers projects to offer an expanded menu of services to members with dementia. The pilot project defined a model of care coordination that included licensed social worker care coordinators, CHWs, volunteers, and a companion model of care and referral relationship with the Alzheimer's Association. To their role, the CHWs brought enthusiasm, interpersonal skills in working with the members and families, knowledge of the community and of how to access agency services, and the capacity to learn their role in the health plan care team.

The team leaders—health plan care coordinator social workers and their colleagues—were able to carve out a role for the CHWs, train and oversee them in that role, find members who could benefit from the additional support, and coordinate the CHW activities with the volunteer and post-diagnosis dementia care initiatives. The study design was not strong enough to determine if the one-third increase in the care coordinators' own caseloads was enabled by the addition of these new service and linkage resources.

The CHW role was terminated with the end of the project. A challenge grant from the California Community Trust was obtained for a larger demonstration of the model, but the matching funds were not found. One of the two remaining CHWs returned to retirement and the other took a related job with KP. While the CHWs ended within KP, the project spurred a broad-based effort to get CHWs for the county through the Community Heath Improvement Partners (CHIP), a collaboration of San Diego health care systems, hospitals, community clinics, insurers, physicians, universities, community benefit organizations, and the County of San Diego.

TEMPORARY DECLINE

The Developers and Their Goals

This project was developed by a geriatrician in the KP Hawaii region. The project's goal was to provide a short period of personal care services at home for health plan members who needed help because of a temporary functional decline due to recent illness or injury, but who did not meet standard skilled care criteria. Health plan goals were to allow safer discharges from the hospital and from skilled home health care in the context of short hospital and skilled home health lengths of stay. It was anticipated that the social goals would be caregiver respite and support. These services were not a part of standard member benefits, and it was important to determine what types of patients would use the benefit and what types of help would prove valuable.

Planning, Development, and Implementation

The 2-year project began with a 6-month development period, followed by an 11-month period in which services were provided, and ending with a 7-month period to gather and interpret the data and to provide a final report. The project was managed by a registered nurse, who determined eligibility, assessed patients' status, oversaw services, and collected project data. Direct services were provided by certified nursing assistants, aides, or both working on contract from the KP home health agency.

The intervention was offered to members who were 18 years or older, who resided within a 12-mile area from Pearl City to Kahala, Hawaii, and who consented to participate in the project. Clinical referral criteria were a recent illness, surgery, or injury that resulted in need for assistance with physical or instrumental activities of daily living, and with functional improvement expected in 2 weeks or less. Additionally, patients had to be largely homebound, not in need of acute hospital-based care, living in a safe home environment, and to have a sound plan of care.

Project enrollment was projected to be between 30 and 70 patients. The project was presented to teams of managed care coordinators, social workers, and rehabilitation in ambulatory care clinics, hospital discharge departments, and the KP home health agency. The ideas did not need much explanation, since staff could readily see appropriate uses. Four data collection sheets were developed covering admitting criteria, intervention, satisfaction, and impact. There was also a certified nursing aide services log and a provider interview data sheet.

Characteristics of Members Served

There were 74 referrals, which resulted in 53 interventions for 51 different patients (two patients were referred twice). Patients for whom interventions were not completed were patients who were referred before staff were ready, did not meet criteria, or declined participation. Eight interventions occurred with patients younger than 65 years old, while 24 occurred with those 65–79, and 21 with those 80 or older. The most common referral conditions were musculoskeletal injury or post-operative recuperation (Table 5.3). Almost all

TABLE 5.3   Primary Diagnosis Leading to Functional Decline and Intervention

Diagnosis	Number of patients
Acute musculoskeletal condition	16
Acute cardiovascular condition, non surgical	5
Neurologic condition/dementia	5
Post operative	12
Pulmonary including pneumonia	7
Infection	4
Advanced cancer	3
Diabetes	1

referrals were for post-hospital care. The hospital-based managed care coordinators quickly became aware of the program and used it enthusiastically. Nine of the patients served came from home health.

The demonstration HSF (completed at this site by the project director) reflects the project's service to members who had recent surgery or hospitalization (Table 5.1). More than 90% had been hospitalized in the previous year; more than 80% had been to the emergency department in the previous 6 months; 62% were taking five or more prescription medications; and 60% reported four or more chronic health conditions. Cognitive dysfunction was rare, but this was not a very mobile group: only 14% could walk stairs; 78% needed help bathing; 34% needed help with 3–5 ADLs; and 58% were using three or more types of adaptive equipment.

Demographically, the HSFs show that the project targeted members who had very weak social support. There was a preponderance of non-married members who were living alone or with children or other relatives; only 16% were married and living with a spouse. Sixty-percent were female. The location in Hawaii is reflected in the high proportions of Asians, Pacific Islanders, and other non-African-American minorities.

Additional project data collection asked who was the primary caregiver: 36% listed a family caregiver who was not a spouse, 19% listed a friend, 17% said a spouse, and 28% had no primary caregiver (8% listed a hired helper). Fully 62% had no live-in caregiver. Many patients were extremely stressed and in difficult situations. Mrs. B was a typical and appropriate case for project services.

Temporary Decline: The Case of Mrs. B

Mrs. B was 51 and had a long history of diabetes and was blind due to diabetic retinopathy. In addition she had peripheral neuropathy, Parkinson syndrome, and carpal tunnel syndrome. She had carpal tunnel release done as an outpatient and was discharged home with a long arm cast. She was divorced and lived with her 13-year old son who had attention deficit hyperactivity disorder with borderline autism. She was not home bound and did not require skilled home care services, so she did not qualify for the standard post-acute home care benefit, but she did need help with managing home activities and her son. She wasn't able to do housework or bathe independently because of the cast. Three home visits were provided to assist with these activities. The cast was subsequently removed, and she returned to managing on her own.

Services Provided

The most common kinds of help were personal care, assistance with mobilization, and homemaking tasks (Table 5.4). The project anticipated that many patients would need up to 20 hours of care. This turned out not to be true. Visits ranged from one to three hours, with an average of 1.5 hours. The average number of visits necessary was two: 10 patients were visited only once, 35 twice, 6 three times, and 2 received five visits.

Making the distinction between services provided as a part of this intervention and services provided via usual home care benefit was not as difficult as anticipated. Most of these patients did not qualify for skilled services under Medicare because (a) although dependent, they were not "homebound" in the Medicare definition, which excludes homeboundness "because of feebleness and insecurity brought on by advancing age"; and (b) they did not require "skilled services," since their service needs could be met without the direct care or supervision of a nurse. Those who had used skilled services still had a period of need for assistance after the need for skilled services resolved.

The project demonstrated a gap in services when services are provided based on staff skills rather than patient needs. The services that were valued were the skills of a trained paraprofessional. Personal care was of more practical importance to these patients than the more narrowly defined medical model of skilled care. The Medicare Home Health Agency Manual states that home health aide services are a covered service only when provided in combination with covered skilled home health services: ". . . *the unavailability of a competent person to provide a nonskilled service, notwithstanding the importance of the service to the patient, does not make it a skilled service. . . .*" Moreover, the types of services delivered by the aides in the project included not only what the manual allows aides to provide in skilled care (e.g., personal care, dressing changes, assistance with medications) but also activities they are not allowed to do under skilled Medicare (general housekeeping, grocery shopping, and meal preparation).

TABLE 5.4   Categories and Types of Services Provided in Temporary Decline Project

General and specific services	Visits in which this service was provided	% of total services provided
Personal Care Hygiene	*44*	24%
Bathing	41	
Perineal care	40	
Skin care	41	
Toe/fingernail care	5	
Mouth care	13	
Shave	11	
Hair care	38	
Dressing	40	
Mobilization Assist	*51*	28%
Ambulation	49	
Transfers	30	
Exercise	4	
Turn and position	5	
Other	1	
Assistance with nursing	*18*	10%
Dressings	4	
PO fluids assist	3	
Medication assist	12	
Nutrition	*23*	12%
Feeding	3	
Meal prep	22	
Homemaking Tasks	*47*	26%
Bed linen change	35	
Dishes	24	
Shopping	15	
House chores	26	
Respite	1	
Total	183	100%

The reason for unexpectedly low utilization was not clear. In some instances, patients appeared to need only a brief period of support and stated that they were getting better and did not need further help. The nine patients who were initially receiving services under skilled home care benefit received some home health aide services during that intervention. Those hours of service provision were not included in project data. Despite shorter than expected episodes, even these services would not have been provided were targeting dependent on skilled home care criteria.

Participant Impact and Feedback

The most recurrent theme in the interviews and questionnaires was that this intervention provided a person not only to care for the patient physically but also emotionally and socially. Patients were frequently anxious about leaving the protected and supported hospital environment when they were still dependent and not well. The intervention provided important follow-up support.

Karnofsky functional score data were collected at the beginning and the end of the intervention and estimated back to baseline before the acute episode (through retrospective reporting by patients). This scale scores individuals from 100 (normal, no complaints, no evidence of disease) to zero (deceased). Most patients in the project scored in the middle ranges: from 50 (requires considerable assistance and frequent medical care), to 60 (requires occasional assistance but is able to care for most needs), to 70 (can care for self but unable to carry on normal activity or do active work). At the time of referral, almost all referrals had declined from their baseline functional status (Table 5.5). At the conclusion of the intervention, many were better but few were back at their baseline functioning before the episode.

A participant survey found that this service filled important needs that would have been difficult for many members to address on their own. When asked if they would have used other help had the project's aide not been available, 20 of 49 respondents said yes, and 19 said no (others weren't sure). Of those who would have looked for other help, most said they would have sought more help from family, friends or neighbors. Six said they would have tried to hire someone. Patients' answers to a question about what they would have done without the health plan aide illustrate the range of needs that were addressed and the barriers that patients faced getting someone else to help them (Box 5.8). When asked to rate the service on a scale of importance, almost all responded "Very important." The most valuable services were personal care (such as bathing), home making, chores, and social support. A letter from a daughter of a patient who received services was typical of family reactions (Box 5.9).

People expressed gratitude for the service and an almost universal willingness to pay a premium for it. They cited their concerns about being unable to do daily life activities and the unavailability of unpaid social support.

Provider Feedback

There was a broad consensus among health plan providers that this intervention helped with patients who were being discharged from the hospital but who had weak social support. Staff felt that it led to safer discharge plans and helped with patients who had social and emotional needs as well as physical needs. Staff viewed these patients as a "gap group" who didn't qualify for

TABLE 5.5 Functional Status Change for Temporary Decline Patients (Karnofsky Scores) (n = 53)

	Baseline before acute episode	Start of intervention	After intervention
Largely independent (70–100)	69%	9%	35%
Needing assistance (51–69)	26%	67%	53%
Dependent (50 or less)	5%	24%	12%
	100%	100%	100%
• Decline of 20 or more from baseline to start of episode:		60%	
• Improvement from start to end of intervention:			
< 10 Karnofsky points		55%	
10–19		30%	
20 or more		6%	

traditional services but who still needed assistance. Staff said that these patients felt better leaving the hospital because there was some follow-up after discharge. Said one, she felt better "just knowing someone was coming from Kaiser."

Assessments of impact on providers themselves were also positive. The project helped physicians and staff feel more comfortable with discharges. One staff member pointed out that the project was a way of getting services

---

BOX 5.8   Temporary Decline Project

"Would your situation be different without this intervention?"

- I can't afford other help.
- I am feeling a whole lot better compared to the first day out of the hospital. I am happy to get this kind of service.
- Zero time off for family and friends for household duties.
- I feel that this should be an included benefit for the people who need it.
- No one around during the day.
- Dependent on neighbors.
- Without service . . . unable to shop and pay utility bills.
- Help was able to prepare ice packs for my foot swelling.
- Laundry wouldn't get done.
- Without help . . . unable to keep casts dry.
- Family help only available after hours.
- It is difficult to find people who are willing to help others because of time involved.
- Wouldn't have the opportunity to get out and ambulate.

BOX 5.9   A Caregiver's Experience with Temporary Decline

After a 17-day hospital stay for pneumonia, my 81-year old mother came home an invalid and we had no idea how to care for her. It was truly a Godsend when we were told she would have a community nurse stop in twice a week for 2 weeks. Nurse Cheryl stopped in the very next day and did an assessment of the home environment, counseling us how to make the home safer. She was also gentle but firm in insisting that my mother use the shower chair. Without her firm insistence, the shower chair would not have become a reality. Now she is able to bathe herself because of this health care aide.

---

into the patients' homes when they otherwise would be resistant. Without this kind of support, these types of patients tended to stay longer in the hospital, since physicians were less willing to discharge. Having the aide to offer also encouraged patients to become more aware of their need for assistance.

Views about the impact on the health plan were positive, but there was less consensus. Several staff felt this program facilitated a shorter hospital stay. Several staff felt it decreased likelihood of hospital readmission. A number felt this was positive for KP's image.

Participating providers almost all wanted the program continued and believed it was worth the funds spent. They also suggested improvements, such as better logistics, including a better liaison, and having the caregiver meet the patient in the hospital. Also, it was not clear who was to define duties for the aide.

Summary

This pilot project identified significant numbers of adults who experienced temporary as well as longer-term functional decline in conjunction with illness or injury, but who would not have been served under usual/Medicare criteria for skilled home health services. Pilot project home health aides working under contract to the KP home health agency provided unskilled support services (e.g., personal care, general housekeeping, and assistance with mobilization) to these "unskilled" but functionally at-risk patients. Demand for the service was strong in terms of willingness to participate but surprisingly short-lived: average visit length was 1.5 hours and mean number of visits was two (maximum five).

Because most patients were socially isolated, direct care was more important than caregiver respite and support as a reason for service. Thirty-three of the 53 interventions occurred in situations in which there was no live-in assistance. But caregiver support was not unimportant: among those patients who lived with a spouse, the spouse was frequently frail. Satisfaction data showed participating patients to be extremely grateful that the health plan would play this role. Almost all expressed willingness to pay extra premiums for the service.

Much larger numbers and a randomized design would be necessary to determine what impact, if any, this type of intervention would have on patient outcomes and cost of care. The extent of utilization if it were to be offered as a covered service is also unknown. In a service area of 200,000 members, the project generated 70 referrals and 53 episodes of care in 11 months. It is suspected that over time, with increased system-wide awareness, non-hospital-based referrals would have increased.

ADAPTIVE EQUIPMENT

The Developers and Their Goals

The Clark County Adaptive Equipment Project in Washington State was proposed by the long-time director of service coordination in the Social HMO, a program which greatly expanded the coverage and use of adaptive equipment and supplies. The project proposed under the Manifesto aimed to improve health plan members' and clinicians' access to assistive technology (AT, also called "adaptive equipment"). The project proposed to educate members and health plan staff about types of AT available and how to obtain it. The ultimate goals were to increase discussion between providers and patients about need for and use of AT, to increase referrals to therapists who could help members decide about purchasing AT and teach them how to use them, and thus to increase the level and appropriateness of utilization. A functional and psychosocial assessment by a medical social worker was available to identify equipment needs and options, and to facilitate referral to appropriate equipment resources.

Planning, Development, and Implementation

The centerpiece of the project was an AT display at the Cascade Park Medical Office in Vancouver, WA, where members, caregivers, and health plan staff could view a wide range of AT not covered by Medicare—from bathtub benches and grab bars to dressing and kitchen aids. Various vendors were contacted to supply items for the display, and one helped to set it up.

An occupational therapist created educational resources for members, caregivers, resource nurses, and clinics to increase awareness and understanding of AT use and availability. KP Northwest region guidelines follow Medicare, which excludes many practical supportive and adaptive items, such as grab bars, bath benches, and bedside commodes. Categorizing these items as a convenience is one of the reasons that a need for them is often overlooked by clinicians and other health plan staff.

A broader plan for internal and external publicity included developing a theme, distributing flyers, and developing TV ads with the help of the health plan's community relations department. The Columbian (Vancouver's major daily newspaper) ran an article on the project, including a picture, and this spurred a letter from the Area Agency on Aging. There were also articles in the KP member quarterly. Project staff met with Independent Living Resources (the local agency for adults with disabilities) and with AARP, which agreed to co-host an open house. All were happy to put their literature at the display. A web site was also created for the final three months of the project, and during that time there were 604 "hits."

There were also efforts to reach members more directly. Two "open houses" were held to increase awareness of the opportunities available to members through this project. There were outside speakers, videos on AT from the University of Buffalo (which has an AT center), refreshments, and prizes. The project's occupational therapist and social worker also went to member meetings. Materials developed included flyers that were posted, a self-referral form, resource lists, posters, and an exam room brochure called "Gizmos, Gadgets and Thingamajigs" (the term "AT" was thought to be a turn-off and not inclusive of such things as zipper helpers). A plan was developed to staff the display, which included social workers, vendors, and volunteers. Throughout the project, the pharmacy showed videos in the waiting area next to the display.

The social worker presented to health plan providers at seven module meetings. She also met with cooperative health care patient groups and COPD (chronic obstructive pulmonary disease) patient groups. The next quarter she met with continuing care nurses, health plan care coordinators, and office nursing staff.

Implementation was somewhat disappointing in terms of using the display as a place to interact with members. Although attractive, the display proved difficult to staff. The project social worker did not have the time to be there except for brief periods. Vendors were not committed and generally did not follow through on commitments to be there. Attempts to find a volunteer to man the display were unsuccessful. By default, two types of staff ended up giving help most often: in their work facilitating referrals, customer services representatives answered questions at the display, and because the display was outside the pharmacy, pharmacists also fielded questions. The spotty staffing made it difficult to know how many members used the display. Many brochures and other materials were taken, but there was no way to evaluate who was taking them or what they did with them.

Open houses were effective in increasing foot traffic and referrals. Even here there were some disappointments, however. AARP would not agree to do a joint event at the health plan open house during AARP's "independent living" month. And again vendors were less available than had been anticipated. Perhaps some of the shortfall was due to timing. Staff concluded that the six weeks they allowed was not enough time to plan such events.

Services Provided

Over 10 months of operations, 34 referrals to the project resulted in social work assessments of need. Two-thirds (23) of the referrals were self referrals, usually based on having seen the display. Provider referrals were from therapists (4), physicians (3), plus one each from social work, nursing, health education, and case management.

After assessment, the social worker tried to connect the member to the source for the AT that was needed. The source generally was either the KP durable medical equipment department or the company that supplied the item. The most frequent types of AT needed were walkers (6 members), bathing aides such as benches or grab bars (6), chair lifts (3), and reachers (3). There were two referrals each for canes, dressing aids, raised toilet seats, kitchen aids, and motorized scooters. There were also one referral each for a transfer aid, a low vision telephone, a binocular magnifier, a car seat, a tailbone cushion, and a ramp or elevator.

Characteristics of Members Served

Twenty-nine of the referred members completed HSFs (Table 5.1). The health and functional status data they reported are somewhat contradictory—on the one hand, relatively high rates of fair to poor health and high rates of health conditions interfering with activities; on the other, relatively low rates of hospital admissions and chronic health conditions. Only 34% needed help bathing, 18% needed help with three or more ADLs, and 36% needed help with four or more IADLs. Compared to the individuals served by most other projects, these were relatively mobile, with 45% being able to walk up a flight of stairs and only 10% using wheelchairs. Perhaps the relatively high rates of health problems and low rates of functional problems were consistent with the targeted nature of the need for AT—e.g., a member could be quite mobile and independent but still use AT to help with vision, reaching, or in the kitchen. Even if they didn't have a condition that interfered with an ADL or mobility, members still had a health condition that affected some activity. The participating members were also a relatively well-connected group socially. Well over half were married and living with a spouse.

Provider and Participant Feedback

This project did not survey or interview either health plan providers or members directly, so project staff used their behavior as indicators. Regarding providers, staff concluded that despite outreach and education efforts, they had not succeeded in making AT an issue that reached the top of many providers' lists. And the weak impact was not just with physicians: health resource centers never asked for videos on subjects such as safe transfers or AT. While physicians made few direct referrals, they did let the project put fliers in waiting rooms, and they did ask the social worker to help accurately fill out forms for obtaining durable medical equipment (DME).

Members seemed easier to reach. The high ratio of self referrals to provider referrals showed that it is possible to educate consumers so that they can advocate for themselves when visiting clinicians. This led project principals to recommend that emphasis be on educating members to ask the physician for a referral. Then the full evaluation would be done after the referral. The presence of AT project materials in waiting rooms may have reinforced the appropriateness of asking.

Lessons

The conceptual model for this project was based on the project director's experience in KP's Social HMO demonstration, which has fostered widespread and successful use of AT among frail Medicare beneficiary members. The expectation was that a prominent display, coupled with referrals from clinicians educated to think about possible AT needs, would increase referrals and utilization. These would be alternative approaches to the Social HMO's service coordinators, who assess frail members in their homes and who can not only recommend but also pay for a wide range of AT not covered by Medicare.

It is not possible to determine if the 34 members referred represented an increase in utilization over what would have happened without the project; but even if all were new users and if all referrals resulted in use of the needed AT, the numbers appear small over a 10-month period. It was difficult to get provider staff, vendor staff, or community partners to engage directly with members who could potentially use AT. It is also not known how much cost entered into the ultimate decision of members to purchase these uncovered services. The transparent access through the display did reach some members, but we don't know the extent to which it helped meet the real extent of need.

The display itself was apparently the single most effective source of self-referrals, even without constant staffing. Back-up help was deemed important, however, and it was recommended that pharmacy staff at each clinic (or membership service personnel) could have a trained, knowledgeable "equipment specialist" with resource information to help members procure DME. This person should also be able to recognize the need for and be able to facilitate therapy referral (by directing the member back to their primary care clinician) so that appropriate equipment could be identified.

Other recommendations for long-term maintenance included putting the project name and a contact name on all materials, always having a mention or article in the monthly newsletter, and not using the term "assistive technology," which members found intimidating and not descriptive.

LESSONS FROM THE PROJECTS

Manifesto 2005 envisioned changing the ways a medical care organization thinks and acts about addressing the needs of its patients with disabilities. The projects in this chapter highlighted the kinds of required internal changes that are implied in this vision. Taken together with the projects discussed in the last two chapters, a set of guideposts to "looking inward" to make the necessary changes to realize the vision begins to emerge (Box 5.10).

Training, Education, and Information

The four cases in this chapter illustrate that, even in a strong and sophisticated system like KP, there were serious shortfalls in consciousness of community care issues and options, as well as in systems to link with community care services. This was borne out most dramatically in the dementia focus group findings about the inadequacy of information and support that members received when first given a dementia diagnosis. Other projects—as well as other studies inside and outside of KP—confirm this "don't ask, don't tell" dynamic that includes, on the one hand, physicians' common reluctance

---

BOX 5.10   Guideposts to "Looking Inward" to Enhance Community Care Linkages
• Get providers and care managers the training and information they need (but no more).   • Accommodate the non-routine in the routine clinic visit.   • Use or create a team that cares about community care.   • Enhance information and tracking systems and use the data to show impacts.   • Extend coverage (just a little).   • Create member-friendly and community agency-friendly contact points, and get feedback from members.

to ask their patients about how they get by in their daily activities, and, on the other hand, patients' reluctance to ask their busy doctors for help with such mundane matters.

All four of these projects, as well as the ones in other chapters, used much the same methods to tell physicians and other providers and care managers about their project and how to use it. They used in-services, prescription pads, handouts, team meetings, individual meetings, and more to get the messages out. They focused on the positive—what providers were doing right rather than doing wrong, and how they could build on those strengths. Assuming that all project leaders and teams made similar efforts, were there any patterns to the successes and failures of internal linkage?

On the one hand, each project found a core of staff who were interested in the projects, readily understood what they were about, took the training, and used educational materials. We have broadly called these "continuing care" staff, and they included social workers, discharge planners, nurse managers, home health, and geriatric groups. It may make sense to have these staff be multiply trained, so that they can handle assessments of multiple dimensions of need and connect members with various kinds of community care resources. More on this below.

On the other hand, it was extremely difficult to reach physicians and affect their behavior. With the exception of a few sites and projects (particularly the dementia project), very few primary care physicians referred their patients to project services. It seemed to be largely beyond the power of project staff to get physicians to regularly engage in discussions about or make referrals to caregiving classes, AT evaluations, volunteer services, adult day services, or the like. The dementia project's apparent exceptions may be due to the fact that physicians get put on the spot in diagnosing dementia and facing member expectations to do something about it. Here a demonstration project folded nicely into a felt need. Small, narrow projects such as assistive technology did not seem to be able to acquire that status unless they were at the top of a particular physician's list (e.g., a geriatrician concerned with continuing care).

These difficulties gaining physician cooperation put on the table the questions of (a) how much effort to put into educating physicians about community care issues, and (b) what to ask them to do. Perhaps what is reasonable is (a) just to train physicians to recognize when there may be problems with function or cognitive status and getting help for problems, (b) to give them some things to ask and say to show their concern, and (c) to get them to refer the patient to someone who can probe further and do something about care needs. In short, consistent with the idea that "your integration is my fragmentation," don't give physicians more information and responsibility than it is reasonable to expect for them to accept. Continuing care staff understood how busy physicians were and also how important it was that they did their primary job of medical care; but they also knew that a timely and confident referral to continuing care could be the key to getting members to accept help, reduce lengths of office visits for complex patients, and also increase their satisfaction.

Fitting the Non-routine in the Routine Office Visit

There may be another support that needs to be added to primary care practice, however, and this is provision for the member who may need a longer or a different type of office visit because of any of a series of cognitive, mobility, community support, or complex chronic illness issues. No specific project in the demonstration addressed this issue, and it really relates to a responsibility of the current medical care system rather than to an extension of the system into community care issues. However, it did come up in the Adult Foster Care project, where one conclusion was that the standard office visit format was inadequate to deal with the needs of many of the participants. Better linkage with community care systems could help ambulatory care prepare for these kinds of needs, as could the types of database analyses that were explored in a project to be described in the next chapter. Another approach is to bring the office visit to the community residents through long-term care physician/nurse practitioner teams, as happens in the foster care pilot that succeeded the demonstration in the Northwest region.

A Linkage Team that Cares about Community Care

The demonstration sites showed that in a clinic-based group model like KP, a number of concerned nursing and social work staffs could see the need to do more to identify patients who need community support and to inform them about community care options and connect them with help. They went by various names in different regions, but they were mostly found doing discharge planning, home health, medical social work, continuing care, and geriatrics. It was these staff who were most prepared to hear about the demonstration leaders' projects, to understand them quickly, and to work out how to connect projects with existing systems and personnel. It was their program infrastructure that was strengthened and extended by the projects.

If a community care linkage system is going to be created, it makes sense to give the lead to these existing staff categories and coordinating structures that already care about and know about community care. In some demonstration sites there were already existing structures (e.g., care coordination teams, member help lines) that could be used, while in others these types of structures were created (and often continued after the end of the projects because they were found useful).

Because these staffs were already on the edge of providing the assessment, care management, and follow-up functions that linkage requires, adding these functions to their jobs was not terribly expensive. But there were real additional costs. Prior to the demonstration, their primary job was to connect members to covered services, and this kept them more than busy. To take on linkage responsibilities, continuing care staff would need administrative and resource support from top management and clinical cooperation from physicians. The linkage model does not ask for a radical makeover from any of these groups or individuals, but the targeted changes in behavior, thinking, and resource use are important to success.

Moving beyond linkage into coordination with community care agencies would require additional capabilities in KP's medical care systems. The Adult Foster Home project discussed in Chapter 4 was perhaps the best example of this. The abnormally high hospital use among foster care residents (compared to matched HMO and Social HMO cohorts) reflected the lack of a proactive plan of care for these chronically ill members. The project found a lack of continuity in primary care and a lack of trained personnel in the foster care settings to report symptom changes. But even if foster care providers were more capable, without the internal point person piloted in the project, they would have no one to call, which would put the medical system on a day-to-day footing.

Information and Tracking Systems

In the last decade, HMOs made tremendous strides in automating management and clinical information systems. Great care and thought and process went into deciding on what to include in these systems and what to exclude, and it is not easy—either politically, operationally, or technologically—to make additions. The demonstration projects showed that information about functional status, family caregiving, and use of non-medical community agency services were not included in these systems, and it was seldom possible to get this information added. This left linkage efforts without a key piece of infrastructure for working successfully with community agencies, following up with members, and alerting the health plan's clinicians about member needs and service utilization. Some projects were able to jury-rig pieces of information and tracking systems, but for the most part hopes in this area were not realized. Because of the complexities of altering information and clinical systems, it is not surprising that this happened, but a linkage model could not go far without progress in this area. Finally, effective use of information to justify what has been done and to show impacts will help build and maintain support for linkage activities.

Coverage Extensions

Community agencies and health providers and care coordinators for frail elders all asked for extensions of service coverage or financing to fill particular holes in benefits that were not being filled by the community. The starting point for adding benefits was to not duplicate anything that already existed in the community or within the health plan. On the community side, agencies wanted back at least modest recognition of the special care they were giving KP members, and in some cases KP did give back (e.g., community benefit grants for volunteers, and the support of health educators in the caregiver training project). Other cases of coverage extensions included KP's own support for volunteers, or more directly the two projects in this chapter that extended coverage of in-home aides beyond Medicare criteria.

Although adding benefits seems like the most dangerous and slippery part of the slope towards new costs, it was remarkable how low-cost these additions were. Almost all projects proved to have lower utilization and demand than anticipated, and thus lower costs. The CHW and temporary decline aides were perhaps most surprising in this regard, since both public and private insurers fear covering such "long-term care." In the Hawaii project, data showed that declines were not always temporary, but patients were still discharged after a maximum of five visits. In the San Diego project, dementia patients served by CHWs had no prospects of their decline being temporary, but services were still not overwhelmed with demands. Members and families were delighted to see the service, but they didn't keep asking for more. KP care managers and clinicians quickly understood the purposes of the services, but they did not use them extensively. Utilization would certainly increase if the projects were made permanent and available more broadly in their regions, but the use of both appeared to be amenable to definition and management. A permanent project would need to continue to be clear about whether to have narrow targeting (e.g., dementia, temporary decline) or something broader (e.g., social isolation/risk).

User-friendly Contact Points

The final component of inner changes suggested by these and the earlier projects is to create user-friendly points of contact for members and community agencies. Because members and agencies have different types of information needs, therefore some projects used different points for each group. Members needed information about what to do to get help to address their needs. This was in some projects a very specialized contact point to get information about how to access a specific service such as caregiver training classes. In others it was more generalized help line—for example, in the form of the San Francisco referral program that could help members think through their needs and then help them connect to any of a variety of options. In either case, the key is to make the way to connect clear, quick, and easy. These information points can also be a vehicle for getting feedback from members about how well the system is working for them.

Community agencies wanted a different type of information. They wanted a place to call to communicate about the status and needs of individual patients. Ideally, the person they would reach in the HMO would know about the type of service the agency provided, the clinical status of the patient about whom they were calling, and even have a personal relationship with the patient. Additionally, to make any of this work, they would have to have a release from the patient to communicate about personal and medical information.

In summary, the internal changes that the health plan needed to make to accommodate the linkage model were not trivial, and they were not free. But they were not illogical, impractical, or perhaps even unaffordable. There were resources in the communities that the these KP regions served that were ready to help its most vulnerable and needy members, and the health plan was able to do things to help members get to those resources. In the process there was clearly a payoff for members and their families, and there was support and reassurance for health plan staff who were charged with sending these members across the border into community care. This demonstration cannot really say whether there was a payback for the health plan itself in terms of reduced service utilization and costs. The question to consider is whether savings should be the standard for deciding whether to invest in a system that could produce these other types of benefits.

REFERENCES

Brown, C. J., Mutran, E. J., et al. (1998). Primary care physicians' knowledge and behavior related to Alzheimer's disease. *Journal of Applied Gerontology, 17*(4), 462–479.

Fortinksy, R. H. (1998). How linked are physicians to community support services for their patients with dementia? *Journal of Applied Gerontology, 17*(4), 480–498.

Leutz, W., Capitman, J., et al. (2001). A limited entitlement for community care: How members use services. *Journal of Aging and Social Policy, 12*(3), 43–64.

6

Infants, Children, and Non-elderly Adults with Disabilities

Carla Green, Nancy Vuckovic, Pauline Bourgeois, Aurora deJesus, Mark Hornbrook, Kathy Brody, and Marlene McKenzie

The Inter-Regional Committee on Aging (IRCOA), as the name implies, was a group focused on improving elder care throughout Kaiser Permanente nation-wide. The IRCOA recognized, however, that older members were not the only ones facing challenges due to impairments in physical and cognitive functioning. For this reason, the committee decided to expand the focus of Manifesto 2005 to include younger members with disabilities. In so doing, the IRCOA has helped to provide a more complete picture of health plan members living with disabilities, how disability varies across the life span, how care needs and informal caregiving functions differ according to life stage and disability, the kinds of community care services and agencies that serve these populations, and the issues that are involved in trying to link and coordinate with those agencies.

Although fewer demonstration projects were related to younger members, they clearly showed parallels to the projects with elders, while also providing new insights. One important difference between this chapter and the others is that all five projects described here included individuals who had mental health disabilities—conditions that can be severely disabling and are more prevalent among younger individuals.

The intent of the first project was to see if it was possible to identify members likely to need special attention because of their disabilities. The project used health plan administrative databases that track applications for short- or long-term disability benefits to try to identify these members. Such information could be used for outreach and intervention, and to make preparations for patients' special requirements during medical office visits.

The next two projects were needs assessments, funded because little was known about the types of services and linkages needed by the children and adults they targeted. The first project used focus groups to study the experiences of parents of children with various disabilities. The discussions identified parents' and children's needs, and made recommendations for how service delivery could be enhanced in response to those needs. The second project used individual interviews to assess needs and recommend home- and community-based care solutions for adults aged 18–64 with one of several disabling conditions characterized by repeated flare-ups: rheumatoid arthritis, systemic lupus erythematosus (lupus), multiple sclerosis, or a serious mental health condition (schizophrenia, schizoaffective disorder, or bipolar disorder).

The fourth and fifth projects were interventions. A Cleveland, Ohio, project linked KP pediatricians with developmental disability-related service providers in state and local agencies to improve care for infants and children who had developmental delays or who were otherwise at risk. The other intervention project arose out of a State of Vermont mandate that Supplemental Security Income (SSI) and Medicaid recipients receive their health care in managed care organizations. The demonstration supported a project to help these new members transition into managed care and to improve the linkages between KP medical care providers and public SSI/Medicaid community care service providers.

Despite large differences in the goals, methods, and populations targeted by these different projects, taken together they can be seen as providing pictures, from different angles, of important care needs and aspects of care provision for individuals with disabilities who are not elderly.

DISABILITY EVENT MODELING, OREGON AND WASHINGTON STATE

The Developers and Their Goals

The project team included the Program Director for Economic and Health Services Research at the Kaiser Permanente Center for Health Research, the Director of Medicare Member Screening for KP, and several KP physicians and physician researchers. The aim of this project was to develop and test computerized identification systems for non-aged persons who were likely to have severe functional impairments and associated high needs for health care use. If feasible, such information could be used for early identification of those needing rehabilitation and assistance in coping with their functional losses or in interfacing with traditional medical care services. Such a system could assure rapid access, improve quality of care, and increase the likelihood of desired outcomes. Lastly, tailoring health care encounters to account for significant functional losses is consistent with Manifesto 2005 goals.

Planning, Development, Implementation, and Member Characteristics

The team used existing HMO data systems to search for indicators of significant disability, choosing the KP Northwest medical information transmittal system (MITS) because it tracks members who have applied for release of medical records to support claims for short- or long-term disability benefits—usually from state Supplemental Security Income (SSI) or federal Social Security Disability Income (SSDI). The study population was defined as members who were enrolled in KP continuously during 1997 and 1998 and who had a disability request processed for federal or state disability or vocational rehabilitation services at any time since the MITS tracking system originated in 1987. These 7,847 individual members (about 2% of the health plan population) were matched on age and sex to a comparison group (7,847) of members without applications for disability benefits. The age distribution of the applicant group was wide: 7% age birth to 12, 5% age 13–19, 24% age 20–44, 53% age 45–64, and 11% age 65 or over. Using health plan administrative, clinical, and utilization files, the project team compared the service use patterns of those with disability requests to use patterns of those without such requests.

Results

The study found that disability requesters had substantially higher service use rates in every service category, as well as higher mortality rates. This was true for all ages and all disability types. The team also found that those with requests were more likely to be eligible for Medicaid or Medicare than the comparison group, which is not surprising since eligibility for SSI and SSDI bring eligibility for Medicaid and Medicare, respectively.

During the two years of observation, those with disability applications had substantially higher mortality rates per 1,000 members per year (14 vs. 3), more total hospitalizations (3,821 vs. 961), more nursing home admissions (399 vs. 34), and more surgeries (9,701 vs. 2,313 inpatient procedures; 2,434 vs. 731 outpatient procedures) than those without such applications. The burden of inpatient hospital days was also much higher in those with applications (1,031 days/1,000 person-years) than in the comparison group

(204 days/1,000 person-years). Over the two years of observation, each disability applicant averaged slightly over two days in the hospital, compared to less than one half day for non-applicants. Almost half the applicant inpatient admissions were for emergencies, and the *total* number of inpatient diagnoses (allowing for more than one diagnosis per admission) was much higher for applicants than for non-applicants (19,251 vs. 3,718). These latter statistics suggest more complications and comorbidities among disability applicants.

Applicants were more likely to have nursing home admissions (252 vs. 27), to spend longer in nursing homes when admitted (3,232 days/1000 population vs. 234 days/1000 population), and were much less likely to be discharged to home or self care (43% vs. 59%). Applicants also had a higher proportion of nursing home discharges to adult foster care (2.8% vs. 0.0%), rehabilitation (4.8% vs. 2.9%), other skilled nursing facilities (13.8% vs. 5.9%), and other hospitals (25% vs. 17.6%).

The project team also interviewed specialists and rehabilitation providers to create a list of disabling conditions that might be used to identify individuals who were functionally disabled but had not applied for disability status. They used this list in a subsequent project that will survey members with these diagnoses to assess their functional status and identify the diagnostic indicators most likely to distinguish those with functional limits. The team expects that the combination of data from disability application requests with diagnostic indicators will identify the majority of health plan members with disabilities.

Summary

The most important lesson learned from this project was that a group of high-need individuals could be readily identified using existing health plan administrative records. The approach was broad in that members of all age groups were included, but it was limited in that it missed many individuals with disabilities who had not applied for disability benefits. Its strength, however, was that it used an easily accessible data source to identify large numbers of individuals with significant health care needs who were at risk of early mortality. Individuals identified using such methods likely represented those with the greatest disability and therefore the greatest need. The wide age range among applicants indicates the need for the medical care system to link to a broad range of age-related community care services.

If intervention programs targeted such individuals first, they could be assured of a population with high rates of needing aid, and later program development could integrate additional members with disabilities who have not applied for disability benefits, but who are identified by other means, e.g., SEEK system screening, KP's 4-item "frailty wheel" screener. Once an identification system was in place, physicians could be assisted to provide better care through modified office visits scheduling, quality of care indicators, outcomes assessment, profiling of their patient panels, and special help to patients in obtaining and maintaining their disability benefits. Projects such as Vermont SSI/Medicaid (described below) suggest that this latter type of help could be an important intervention point. In short, the medical system could be anticipating the predictable needs of patients and striving for a centralized care plan area where aspects of significance could be noted and kept up-to-date by all providers and clinical staff.

PARENTS OF CHILDREN WITH DISABILITIES, DENVER, COLORADO

The Developers and Their Goals

The project team was composed of the Medicaid Management Analyst, the Director of Senior Programs for Kaiser Permanente, and the Research Project Coordinator for Senior Programs. The purpose of the project was to study the needs and experiences of parents of children with physical or mental disabilities, and to recommend how service delivery could be enhanced in response to those needs.

Member Characteristics, Implementation, and Study Findings

The project team conducted four focus groups with 25 parents whose children ranged in age from 18 months to 16 years, most (66%) age 6 and younger. The children's conditions included Down Syndrome, cerebral palsy, quadriplegia, hydrocephalus and hemiparesis, cleft lip and palate, cranial stenosis, asthma, spina bifida, premature birth, multiple congenital anomalies, autism, leukemia, microcephaly, and Gullian-Barre syndrome. Indications of their care needs, as reported by their parents on a modified version of the demonstration HSF, appear in Table 6.1. Parents rated their children's health as "fair" or "poor" 45% of the time, and reported that health conditions affected activities for 46% of their children. Many participating children had recent hospitalizations (37%) and ER visits (34%), and although 75% had only three or fewer health conditions, 17% had 4–6 and 8% had 7 or more significant problems. Only 29% of children were free of ADL and IADL limitations. Similarly, 29% needed a wheelchair.

Despite the wide variety of disabilities represented, parental needs were remarkably similar, as evidenced by the quotes in Box 6.1. These needs fell into three categories: (a) information needs, (b) medical care access and continuity, and (c) community care access and benefits.

TABLE 6.1 Participant Characteristics

	Denver Children ($n = 24$)	Ohio Children ($n = 84$)	Vermont SSI ($n = 245$)	Adults with Disabilities ($n = 83$)
Health condition				
Parent-rated health fair or poor	45%	25%	na	33%
Takes 5 or more prescription drugs	4%	6%	na	40%
Health conditions affect activities	46%	54%	na	64%
One or more hospitalizations in last year	37%	33%	31%	29%
One or more ER visits in last 6 months	34%	34%	33%	25%
Reports 0–3 health conditions[a]	75%	72%	52%	na
Reports 4–6 health conditions	17%	23%	23%	na
Reports 7 or more health conditions	8%	5%	25%	na
ADL & IADL[b]				
Does not need help with ADLs	29%	26%	87%	92%
Needs help with 1–2 ADLs	25%	20%	9%	na
Needs help with 3–5 ADLs	46%	54%	4%	na
Does not need help with IADLs	29%	34%	50%	na
Needs help with 1–4 IADLs	71%	55%	36%	na
Needs help with all IADLs	0%	11%	14%	na
Mobility				
Uses a wheelchair	29%	39%	3%	13%
Equipment[c]				
None	46%	26%	76%	na
1–3	46%	56%	21%	na
4 or more	8%	18%	3%	na

TABLE 6.1 (*Continued*)

	Denver Children (n = 24)	Ohio Children (n = 84)	Vermont SSI (n = 245)	Adults with Disabilities (n = 83)
Treatments[d]				
None	4%	75%	91%	na
1–3	50%	21%	9%	na
4 or more	46%	4%	0%	na
Race				
White	na	65%	na	na
Black or African American	na	32%	na	na
Asian or Pacific Islander	na	3%	na	na
Other	na	0%	na	na
(Hispanic origin)	27%	8%	na	na

[a] *Denver & OH:* Diabetes, high blood pressure, heart problems, lung problems, cancer, stomach problems, urinary problems, vision, hearing, mental retardation, cystic fibrosis, eating or feeding disorders, behavioral problems, speech disorders, spina bifida, seizure disorders. *Vermont:* Categories are 0–3, 4–5, 6 or more. Items include: Alcoholism, arthritis, asthma, bad back, bipolar disorder, blind, cancer, cerebral palsy, cystic fibrosis, deaf, other hearing impairment, depression, diabetes, drug dependence, emphysema, epilepsy/seizure head injury, heart disease, high blood pressure, HIV/AIDS, lung disease, mental retardation, migraine headaches, muscular dystrophy, multiple sclerosis, renal/kidney disease, schizophrenia, sickle cell anemia, spina bifida, spinal cord injury, stroke, ulcers, other.

[b] ADLs include bathing including sponge, dressing, using the toilet, getting in/out of bed or chairs, and eating. *Vermont* includes walking, so top group is 3–6. IADLs include doing routine household tasks, managing money, taking medications, transportation, and using the telephone. Vermont also includes shopping for groceries, and preparing meals. So top category is 5–7. *Adults* reported yes/no on ADL limitations.

[c] *Ohio:* Wheelchair, walker, cane, grab bars, bath bench, Hoyer lift, bedside commode, hospital bed, ramps, oxygen equipment, hearing aid, leg braces, crutches. Denver: same as Ohio but no crutches. Vermont has TTY, communication device, wheelchair, walker, cane, grab bars, bath bench, Hoyer lift, bedside commode, ramps, oxygen equipment, other.

[d] Oxygen, aerosol treatment, postural drainage, tube feedings (nose, mouth, or stomach), tracheostomy care, catheter care, colostomy, Broviac/Hickman, decubitus care, frequent suctioning, injections, chemotherapy, occupational therapy, physical therapy, speech therapy, other.

BOX 6.1   Needs of Parents of Children with Disabilities

Information needs
Parents want direction and guidance on what they need to learn and how to go about learning
"You totally have to educate yourself and look at things. Because you don't have any direction, you're kinda going on your own."

"I look at all this information that's out there and ask why is there not a better book or some kind of guidance being offered on this?"

Information about resources is not offered
"It's just helpful to know what's out there. If you don't know what's out there you don't even know what you can access. Honestly, it's hit or miss those first few years."

"They could tell us they can't help but they know somebody else who can help. And then help us get there. You know, not say 'here's the number,' walk away."

Medical care access and continuity
Parents need someone to actively help them get linked, navigate Kaiser system
"Maybe someone could sit down with you and go over your plan and say 'here's what yours covers.'"

"Maybe some sort of liaison to social worker whose job is really to help special needs parents. A number that you could always call and there's someone who can be a liaison with you and outside services or you and your doctor."

Parents want providers to communicate with each other and coordinate care
"It's like nobody knows what's going on. I wish you could have people who specialize in a group and then they get together once a month and talk about your cases. Because nobody knows what anybody else is doing."

Families want to see the same provider when they come to the medical office
"We're not going to walk in and see any doctor that's there because they just sit there and scratch their heads because they don't know her whole background."

"I rarely get to see his primary care doctor. Why can't I see the same person?"

Families want to spend more time with their physicians
"I think they should allow more time for these doctors to have a little bit more one-to-one with these patients and their families."

"I just don't feel like I can call and talk to him on the phone. I mean I get transferred 32 times and then someone takes a message."

BOX 6.1 *(Continued)*

Community care access and benefits
Parents gain support and learn from each other
"It helps to be involved in local support groups."

"Through parent networking is probably where I've learned the most."

Home health visits provide support and reassurance
"Kaiser sent a visiting nurse out and that just totally reassured me. That was so helpful."

"It was so supportive and reassuring. Just having someone with expertise coming into the home."

Parents want a more extensive therapy/DME benefit
"These kids really do have a need medically to continue therapy longer than say someone who's been in a car accident. And I get the feeling that the therapy benefit is really more oriented towards short-term adult problems."

"The $2000 DME cost is a problem; $2000 is a drop in the bucket when you're talking about a $10,000 motorized wheelchair."

Parents wanted to learn more about their children's conditions, wanted assistance with where to find good information, and wanted help in navigating the HMO system. They also needed information about available services within KP and the community, and help linking to those services. Parents' medical care concerns centered around access to KP services and provider knowledge about their children's conditions. Parents felt that they had to really push to get what they needed in terms of information and services—that there was no systematic way of providing or coordinating such offerings by the health plan. They wanted care providers to share more information with each other to better coordinate care, and they wanted their children to be seen consistently by the same health care providers so that these providers would know their children's history and medical needs. Parents also felt a need for longer visits with their health care providers than were typically scheduled.

Community care access and benefits concerns revolved around issues related to home health nurses and support groups for parents. Parents welcomed the support and information gained from other parents of children with disabilities, and found support groups helpful. They also found home health nurse visits supportive and reassuring, wanted information about other types of home health services that might be available, and needed help arranging those services.

Parents perceived that the HMO's staff were not knowledgeable about available health plan and community benefits, and also felt that benefit levels were not adequate: Therapies did not last long enough and the durable medical equipment the health plan provided did not adequately meet needs.

In response to concerns and needs identified in the course of the project, the team made the following recommendations to the health plan:

- Train health care providers to give information about internal and external resources and benefits.
- Work to proactively share information on diagnoses and community benefits.
- Link parents early with a care/service coordinator to do internal and external linkage.
- Improve MD/specialist links.
- Increase length of appointment times.
- Make home health available for emotional support as well as medical conditions.
- Offer support groups to address emotional needs of parents.
- Evaluate adequacy of therapy/durable medical equipment benefit packages.

In order to facilitate system change in response to these recommendations, the project team members implemented several strategies. First, they provided results of the focus group interviews to an existing primary care leadership team composed of the operations chief for Primary Care, the medical operations director and leaders from the Internal Medicine, Family Practice, and Pediatrics departments—a group whose general responsibility is to develop strategic plans for care delivery throughout the region. The primary care leadership team felt that the needs identified by the project were consistent with the problems they had already been addressing in delivery of primary care, and that recently implemented initiatives, such as the designation of Chronic Special Needs Nurses, could be used to address many of the issues raised by parents.

The second strategy to facilitate implementation involved providing results to an ongoing project designed to help managed care organizations develop internal structures and processes to strengthen the care coordination system and build linkages between the HMOs and community-based providers that serve children with special needs who have Medicaid coverage. This program (Safety-Net), funded by the Robert Wood Johnson Foundation, was underway at the time the results of the Denver Parents project became available, so results were presented at a regular Safety-Net project meeting and to the Medicaid and KP coordinators of the project. Findings were used to develop educational sessions and screening tools for the project.

The Denver Parents project also presented their findings and recommendations to the chronic special needs nurses' leadership team, to four nurses designated to address the needs of the pediatric population, and to the director of Perinatal Homecare, which coordinates care for children who require complex home-based services.

Unfortunately, despite efforts to disseminate findings and recommendations from the project, there was no demonstrated change in the delivery of care beyond those described above. There are multiple reasons for this. First, and most importantly, system change was not a goal of this short project, which aimed only to study what changes were needed rather than to implement changes. Second, the project recommendations involved two basic themes—system change and provider training/increased responsibilities—both of which are notoriously difficult to implement without a responsible party who can facilitate such processes. Third, there was no effort to create new linkages with community care resources. The Vermont Medicaid project (described below) provides an example of how a person in a facilitator role can affect care provision at all levels, and can help provide the kinds of linkages and information these parents needed without increasing burden on health care providers. Lastly, projects which were successful in implementing system changes had physician champions who worked to implement key system changes. The absence of such an advocate may have limited the impact of what *might* have been useful information gained by the project. In short, the project confirms that good study and recommendations are not enough to create change. There need to be implementation plans and leadership to follow through.

Summary

Parents of children with disabilities of all types had important needs for information. They wanted to know more about their children's health, about what services were available to help them and their children, and how to access those services. Providing such information could empower parents to find and manage services on their own and to feel more in control of their lives. Parents also wanted their children's health care providers to talk with each other, and they wanted (and needed) more therapy and durable medical equipment benefits than were being offered. This project showed, however, that identifying such needs and informing key stakeholders did not necessarily result in changes that addressed those needs. The lack of change resulting from merely giving out information helps to put in context the achievements of the more intensive linkage and coordination projects described in Chapters 3–5 and later in this chapter.

NORTHWEST ADULTS WITH DISABILITIES, OREGON/WASHINGTON

The Developers and Their Goals

The project team consisted of two researchers from the Kaiser Permanente Center for Health Research—a medical anthropologist and a sociologist—and a health behavior specialist who worked as an interviewer and project administrator. The aim of the Northwest Adults with Disabilities study was to assess the needs of non-elderly adults diagnosed with disabilities likely to produce unpredictable variations in needs for care and support resulting from health conditions characterized by relapses, deterioration, or both.

Member Characteristics, Implementation, and Study Findings

The study team completed interviews with 83 KPNW members (aged 18–64) who had sustained (one year or more) diagnoses of lupus, rheumatoid arthritis, multiple sclerosis, bipolar disorder, schizoaffective disorder, or schizophrenia. These diagnoses were chosen because many non-elderly individuals with these conditions were thought likely to have community care needs yet, with the exception of those who qualify for disability income or Medicaid, few became linked to such care. In the context of Manifesto 2005, individuals with such conditions were thought to be among the strongest candidates for inclusion in community care program expansions.

All groups had significant functional limitations and needs for care (see Tables 6.1 and 6.2). Those with mental health problems also had very poor physical health, and those with multiple sclerosis and lupus had worse mental health in addition to their physical health problems. Overall, all groups had significant physical and social functioning limitations, and all but the group with rheumatoid arthritis had emotional functioning limitations. Participants reported that their health was "fair" or "poor" 33% of the time; 40% took five or more prescription medications each day, and 64% reported that their physical or mental health conditions affected their ability to engage in regular activities. Hospitalizations were common—29% in the last year—as were ER visits in the last six months (25%). Additionally, 8% had ADL limitations, only 52% could walk up one flight of stairs, and 13% needed a wheelchair.

Despite the differences underlying members' needs, the needs were fairly similar across groups. Needs increased during flare-ups, and the participants were most often assisted by informal caregivers. A few participants received disability income, and some of these individuals also received community care services through their Medicaid or Medicare coverage. This was the exception rather than the rule, however, and often such services were limited

TABLE 6.2 Means, standard deviations, and results of t-tests for differences between SF-36 scale scores measuring functioning, and 1998 U.S. general population means.[a] U.S. population norms for each measure = 50; means below 50 indicate health and functional status below population means; asterisks indicate statistically significant differences from these population means.

SF-36 V2. Scale Scores	Schizophrenia or Schizoaffective Disorder[b] M (SD), t	Bipolar Disorder[c] M (SD), t	Multiple Sclerosis[d] M (SD), t	Rheumatoid Arthritis[e] M (SD), t	Lupus[f] M (SD), t
General Health	35.55(9.63), 5.80***	40.69(11.55), 3.01**	38.57(10.99), 4.41***	40.70(8.66), 4.54***	37.45(13.02), 3.83***
Physical Functioning	38.16(13.38), 3.42***	47.57(9.72), 0.93 n.s.	35.62(15.25), 4.00***	36.18(10.36), 5.65***	46.25(7.90), 1.89*
Bodily Pain	45.26(12.13), 1.51+	45.48(11.26), 1.50+	45.68(11.49), 1.59+	40.61(11.41), 3.49***	44.22(9.33), 2.47**
Role-Physical	39.64(14.33), 2.80**	42.04(10.97), 2.71**	36.87(12.01), 4.63***	38.42(12.97), 3.78***	44.44(7.02), 3.06**
Vitality	39.71(9.41), 4.23***	40.35(8.49), 4.24***	39.20(9.3), 4.92***	41.22(11.93), 3.12**	45.00(6.86), 2.91**
Physical Component Summary Score	41.04(14.17), 2.36**	46.77(10.79), 1.12 n.s.	36.83(13.69), 3.96***	35.26(10.10), 6.00***	44.19(7.64), 2.94**
Mental Health	38.32(13.18), 3.43***	38.71(8.6), 4.90***	45.65(10.14), 1.82*	47.92(11.53), 0.76 n.s.	49.03(7.07), 0.55 n.s.
Role-Emotional	34.69(16.69), 3.43***	39.45(12.72), 3.10***	44.78(11.44), 1.88*	48.49(13.12), 0.47 n.s.	44.89(9.57), 2.13*
Social Functioning	39.63(13.62), 2.94**	35.00(11.14), 5.03***	37.81(14.85), 3.48***	42.50(14.48), 2.20*	46.32(8.41), 1.75*
Mental Component Summary Score	35.89(17.90), 2.95**	35.76(11.5), 4.63***	45.33(11.11), 1.73*	50.21(12.92), 0.07 n.s.	46.97(8.66), 1.35+

[a] significance levels for t tests: + $p < .10$, * $p < .05$, ** $p < .01$, *** $p < .001$.
[b] $n = 15$ except for role-emotional, mental component summary score, and physical component summary score where $n = 14$.
[c] $n = 14$.
[d] $n = 16$.
[e] $n = 18$ except for role-emotional, mental component summary score, and physical component summary score where $n = 17$.
[f] $n = 16$ except for role-physical, mental component summary score, and physical component summary score where $n = 15$.

to transportation. Interestingly, two of the participants included in the study because of their mental health conditions received disability income and services because of *physical* health problems.

Consistent with the community care needs of elderly individuals, these adults with disabilities often needed help with housekeeping, meal preparation, transportation, social isolation, medication management/administration, and symptom monitoring. Different from the elderly persons, these younger adults needed additional services, such as child care, but needed other community care services less consistently. Additionally, as expected, needs varied significantly in all groups over time. Some individuals needed care only during flare-ups, while others needed ongoing care, but had additional needs when their symptoms worsened.

Notwithstanding their significant needs for community care, most of the members interviewed did not receive these types of services, or even know they existed; the few who did receive services had Medicare or Medicaid coverage that paid for that care. This points to one of the major findings of this study. As expected, many of these individuals had needs for community care and did not receive it, but the reasons for the lack of care were complicated. First, most were living successfully in the community, supported by informal caregivers. The project team speculated that these individuals had not needed to apply for disability status because of their success at community living, and had few contacts with service agencies because of their informal support systems. Such factors were likely to keep the health plan and health care providers from recognizing the extent of these individuals' needs, so efforts to connect them to community agencies may not have been made. They also point to the potential risks associated with caregiver loss or burnout, as well as the potential importance of linking to services while people are still successful at community living. The following findings illustrate these points.

The care needs of study participants were almost always provided for by informal caregivers, but these caregivers were limited in number (usually 1–2), and many participants worried about their ability to live independently if these care providers were lost. With the exception of support groups, few knew about or received community care services, and those who did know about or receive services were the most severely disabled of the members interviewed. Even though informal care was the norm, it was not always adequate. Sometimes caregivers could not adequately provide care, and sometimes no caregivers were available at all. Indeed, many participants reported social isolation, raising additional concerns about continued independent living if caregivers were no longer able to provide support. Moreover, some study participants were caregivers themselves, further complicating the picture of these interactions. Thus, as is true for many elderly people, interdependent caregiving relationships supported the continued independent living of two individuals with significant functional limitations. Participants' comments, listed in Box 6.2, illustrate these themes and the similarities across participants with varying conditions.

The project team made several recommendations:

- Work to educate individuals with disabilities who have relapsing conditions about available home and community-based care options, and link them to agencies that provide such care.
- Work to educate the health plan and health care providers about the home and community-based care needs of individuals with relapsing conditions.
- Work with existing community-based care organizations to develop methods for providing services during acute exacerbations or when informal support is unavailable, particularly housekeeping, meal preparation, transportation, money management, medication management/administration, and child care.
- Make services available for brief periods, on short notice, with a single point of contact and pre-certification prior to need.
- Help individuals with disabilities expand networks of informal caregivers—family, friends, neighbors.
- Use support groups (composed of individuals at similar functional levels) to expand caregiving networks and reduce social isolation.
- Supplement natural support systems with community visits or call services.
- Evaluate and change benefits and eligibility criteria to adequately address the unmet community care needs of individuals with relapsing conditions.

The results of this project suggest that formal community care programs could be modified to address the needs of individuals with relapsing conditions—providing ongoing care for those who need it, and sporadic care for those who require only periodic assistance or need to supplement regular care. Such a program would have to respond quickly to calls for support, suggesting a pre-certification process and a single point of contact to arrange care when needs arise. In some cases (e.g., for those who live alone, provide care for others, or have severe mental health problems), regular monitoring could be used to supplement informal caregivers, ensuring that individuals needing help are identified early in the flare-up process.

Additionally, social isolation was a significant problem for many of these individuals. Community- or health-plan-coordinated support groups might alleviate some of these social needs as well as increase the pool of informal caregivers and symptom monitors available to individuals. It is important,

BOX 6.2   Comments from Northwest Adults with Disabilities Study Participants

Coping strategies during flare-ups

(participant with schizophrenia) I go into my head. It's more of just a concentration or I get a lot of sleep if I'm not feeling well, I take a certain medicine and I sleep for two or three days and then when I wake up and get back up, then I'm back at a level point.

(participant with multiple sclerosis) If I'm tired when I get up in the morning, then I know it's not gonna be a real good day and I more-or-less don't plan anything for that day. I don't plan to do any heavy housekeeping or going very many places. In fact, on those days I usually stay home and do pretty much nothing all day.

Independence, sheer effort and obligations as motivators for getting through

(participant with lupus) I may be ill, but I still can be independent.

(participant with schizoaffective disorder) Yeah, when I get depressed, I don't want to go to the store. I don't want to do anything with my daughter, you know, but I can't say no. [So you get there anyway?] I get there anyway, yeah.

Key support persons

(participant with schizophrenia) [What do you do about things like eating {when you need to sleep for 2–3 days}?]. My parents basically take care of that.

(participant with lupus) Oh, [my son] doesn't do much physical, but sometimes he'd, you know, fix me like some breakfast, or stuff like that. He drove me to the doctor a couple of times, or drove me to the emergency room. [My daughter] more is, you know, housecleaning when she's here. Cooking meals, stuff.

Concerns about loss of support persons

(participant with schizophrenia) I've had concerns about that [brother and sister-in-law dying] lately. [pause] Yeah. I'd probably have a tough time without them, so I've been kind of worried and stuff. Yeah. They give me a lot of tender, loving care, which is very helpful.

(participant with multiple sclerosis) I would be devastated if something happened to my caregiver, my husband, my friend, my everything. That is a concern, you know. And that's scary.

Difficulty coping without support persons

(participant with bipolar disorder) It was hard to go shopping. I'd run out of food and, you know, like be splitting a package of Top Raman into two meals to put off having to go to the store. [Laugh] And the diet was bad.

(participant with rheumatoid arthritis) [from post-interview notes] In terms of worries about the future, she said that they relate to the fact that she was a single woman, and she had some concerns about being alone in the future and being able to fend for herself.

however, to match needs of the member to the type of support group. Several participants reported attempts to attend support groups, but found that those groups were ill-matched to their needs (e.g., individuals with recent diagnoses of multiple sclerosis attending groups composed primarily of individuals who had mobility impairments that required use of a wheelchair; attendance at a group for individuals with lupus in which most individuals died within one year). Rather than providing support and hope, most participants who reported attending support groups found that they were depressing. A strong exception to this was a community socialization group attended by a participant with a mental health condition, who found great support among the group's members and was able to activate and marshal that support in ways that helped her make it through the roughest times without hospitalization.

Summary

Non-elderly adults with relapsing conditions, whether mental or physical, had significant needs for home- and community-based care. Many of these needs (housekeeping, meal preparation, transportation, and child care) could have been provided for with slight modifications of existing community-based care programs. Pre-certification, allowing provision of services on short notice, and a single point-of-contact to arrange such services, would increase the chance of meeting the needs in this population. Social needs were also critical, but less easily met. Facilitating support groups, matched to participants' functional levels, would be a valuable first step to address the isolation of many of these individuals, and could increase informal caregiving opportunities.

LINKING INFANTS AND CHILDREN, OHIO

The Developer and Her Goals

The project developer was a pediatrician in the Department of Pediatrics and Adolescent Medicine in Cuyahoga County Ohio Kaiser Permanente, and chief consultant for the Ohio region regarding disabilities and special needs. Her position gave her a unique perspective on the status of medical care linkages to community care services, and her status in the region gave her standing with other pediatricians on these issues. The goal of this project was to improve the care and quality of life of special needs children by linking KP primary care pediatric practices with two community and home-based care programs to deliver organized and coordinated services.

Planning, Development, Implementation, and Members Served

The two programs targeted for improved linkage—the Early Intervention Program (EIP) and the County Board of Mental Retardation and Developmental Disabilities (MRDD)—served Cuyahoga County, Ohio, and were located in Cleveland, the county's largest city. KP had 18 pediatricians and three nurse practitioners who provided pediatric primary care in five different facilities in this county, but these practices were not well linked to the community programs targeted. These programs, the EIP and County Board of MRDD, had extensive outreach programs, did home visits, assessed child and family needs, developed the child's individual family service plan (IFSP), shared recommendations with referring physicians, and provided services irrespective of economic status.

Parents were eager to have their children participate in the health plan's project, which enrolled 84 children in the fall of 1998. Children ranged in age from 1 to 18 years; 40% were of preschool age, and 60% were of school age. Rapid enrollment in the program likely reflected one of the study's primary findings—that children needed additional services. They often lacked health care coverage for long-term therapies, durable medical equipment, special nutrition, and home nursing support when parents were working.

Table 6.1 summarizes children's health status and needs, reported by their parents. Of these children, 25% had "fair" or "poor" health, and 54% had health conditions that affected their abilities to engage in routine activities. Hospitalizations (33% in the last year) and ER visits (34% in the last 6 months) were common, and 28% reported having more than three serious health conditions. Only 26% of children did *not* need help with ADLs, while 34% had no need for IADL help. At the same time, 39% used a wheelchair, and the majority used some kind of durable medical equipment (74%).

Project staff learned early on that KP's primary health care providers had limited knowledge of the community agencies, their roles and services, and how to access them. Making matters worse, some community program staffs were skeptical about the HMO's motives. To address these problems, the project director took various approaches, beginning with background research to learn about the services provided by the community care agencies. Second, the director hired a coordinator to facilitate exchange between all organizations involved. Third, she called program directors, visited programs, and involved staff, including the principals, child psychologists, nurses, and therapists from two public schools. In addition, several meetings were held to educate all concerned parties about the goals, services, and expertise of each organization, and to try to begin establishing trust, understanding, and respect for the roles of individuals in each organization.

The community agency meetings allowed staffs from stakeholding organizations to raise and answer questions. Staff members of the community programs were initially skeptical about the motives of the HMO—their impressions were that KP refused services. Strategies were implemented to establish trust and respect for each other's roles and to improve communications and access. Learning about the scope and limits of services on each side fostered trust, and in the end, communications improved and the agencies exchanged referral forms and telephone and fax numbers with KP outreach staff. Agencies were interested in learning about what KP could and could not cover in ongoing therapies. Interestingly, the project team found that clear "no" answers from KP were almost as good as affirmative answers, since established boundaries allowed staffs to begin tapping other resources. The project also facilitated access and better communications with primary care providers (PCPs) for community service agencies.

Despite these efforts, there were few new referrals in the first seven months of the project. To understand why, the project team surveyed PCPs. They still found very poor knowledge of the agencies and their associated services, even though the project had conducted an in-service training and distributed written information, flyers, and program brochures to all appropriate providers. Since these efforts did not produce the intended outcomes—better linkage and greater referrals to the community organizations—the project team decided to take a different approach. They developed an internal linkage to facilitate the education and referral process, using facility-based teams. The facility teams, consisting of pediatricians, a registered nurse, their direct supports, and licensed practical nurses or medical assistants in each medical office, met every two weeks for 60–90 minutes. Targeting this team finally produced the desired system changes. For example, the team reviewed referral forms and suggested that they should be filled out before patients left the office. Once these processes were in place, front-line providers started to see results and became enthusiastic.

These meetings plus the pediatric outreach made a difference. Formerly, the social worker linked with community care if a pediatrician asked, but this didn't lead to broad-based connections. After the training, medical office staff from the teams started calling agencies directly. They learned the criteria for the agencies and felt free to call. People learned that there were four or five agency options, not just one. Feedback from community agencies was that there were more referrals and earlier referrals, which was key in early intervention. The regional early intervention coordinator also reported that more pediatricians were referring directly and at younger ages: In 1999 there were EIP referrals from nine different pediatricians, whereas previously all referrals had come through the project director in her role as special needs consultant. The referral numbers support participants' reports of change. Despite decreasing numbers of deliveries, the number of referrals increased: in Cuyahoga County in 1997 (before the project), KP referred only 12 babies of 1592 deliveries (0.75%). In 1998, 21 of 1,499 were referred (1.4%), and in 1999, 24 of 1,353 babies were referred (1.77%). Toward the end of the project, the project director was asked to sit on the regional early intervention advisory committee, where there was talk of asking other HMOs to set up similar projects.

The Linking Children project also helped with benefit coordination. KP started receiving assessments from the agencies, which allowed medical staff to see what community care was covering. This helped the project director to go elsewhere—out of county or state—for services, and she also began attaching these assessments to facilitate approval of applications for government coverage. The outside assessments became part of the chart, which helped organize needed information in one central location that could be easily sent when needed. In this way, two-way communication helped staff obtain valuable physical and occupational therapy resources for members.

Other resources were also accessed. These included a waiver program giving 20–30 hours a week of home nursing (three project children qualified in 1998, two in 1999), and a program through the Bureau of Children with Medical Handicaps that gave unlimited physical, speech, and occupational therapy for all the children accepted (seven project children qualified in 1998, 10 in 1999). Additionally, the latter program provided orthotics and equipment for five project children. According to the project director, KP providers "now know how to apply to the Bureau to get payment for therapy from other sources. We know the criteria and who qualifies." This project provided important evidence that getting into the community can identify real resources for members, and it taught providers how to access them.

Participant Feedback

Participants also felt the project had been very successful, as can be seen from the following excerpt from a letter sent by a participant to Kaiser Permanente Customer Relations:

> My son has been under the care of (names doctors from project team) and their amazing nurses (names of project nurses). Together these women have provided us with the personalized type of services we all hope to receive but seldom do anymore. Their knowledge of the community resources has made a tremendous difference in the care of my son. We are better able to cope now, having all these services available whenever needed even just for reassurance and stress relief after a particularly frustrating day. This teamwork of the doctors and nurses and the therapists of the community agencies embodies what good medicine should be about— always focusing on the total needs of patients. The medical offices are able to share their medical knowledge with the staff of the other agency that my son attends. Everybody has been very sensitive to the difficulties families experience when trying to make medical decisions, and have always treated us as full partners in the care of our child.

Summary

One of the most important lessons from this project was that it took real resources and actions (not just educational efforts), to get results and that it was *results* that produced the buy-in of busy front-line health care providers. A critical part of the action was to get out into the community to find out about community care resources and to put health care providers, administrators, and the medical care system on the line in terms of promising collaboration. Additionally, continued discussion and teaching at the team level in the medical office, with regular update meetings with community programs, was necessary to maintain gains of this and similar efforts. Lastly, having a committed and well-placed champion of system change facilitated all of these processes.

Other important lessons were that before the project PCPs knew little about what community care programs provided or how to access those services, and community care providers knew little about how health plans worked or what was covered, and were suspicious of their motives. These problems could be overcome with increased communications and a commitment from the HMO to dedicate resources to facilitating the link between the health plan and community care organizations.

Lastly, the project inadvertently learned that this group of children is at high risk of losing coverage. When KP had to raise premiums, about 10 percent of the health plan population disenrolled, while 25 members of the study population lost their KP coverage. The disruptions in coverage and providers that are becoming increasingly common in U.S. health insurance systems are particularly difficult for families and individuals with disabilities. The change of one provider can upset a carefully constructed team working across system borders. The need for continuity lends support to the larger system reforms proposed in Chapter 8.

VERMONT SSI/MEDICAID PROJECT

The Developers and Their Goals

The project developer was the Administrator of Care Management for KP Northeast, and the team included a social worker in the role of Coordinator. This project's primary aim was to establish systems and procedures to successfully enroll and serve SSI/Medicaid beneficiaries transitioning, by state requirement, from Medicaid fee-for-service into KP Vermont. Beneficiaries had the choice of enrolling in KP or another HMO run by Blue Cross/Blue Shield. Project developers hoped to achieve successful transitions by creating working relationships with all groups providing medical care and social services to these recipients.

Planning and Development

Three thousand beneficiaries were expected to move into the KP system, including many with mental illnesses diagnoses and adults with physical disabilities. The SSI enrollment mandate excluded elders, those in nursing homes, those with dual eligibility (Medicaid and Medicare), and adults and children with mental retardation or developmental disabilities.

The specific goals of the project were (a) to reduce fragmentation and duplication by better linking medical offices with behavioral health care providers, community mental health centers, and other community-based agencies; (b) to conduct regular educational and problem-solving meetings with state agencies, community-based agencies, providers, contractors, and advocacy groups representing various disability groups; and (c) to develop a list of resources and services available for this population to be used by providers, case managers, and social workers.

To do this, the project hired an experienced social worker for the new position of "coordinator." The coordinator had responsibility for facilitating links among those providing care for individual enrollees, implementing a triage system for new enrollees (and its associated data systems), organizing meetings between service providers of all types (including medical providers), and managing trainings about KP for community agency staff.

Enrollment began in only two counties to allow participating HMOs time to prepare and test enrollment and service systems. Unfortunately, just a few months into implementation, enrollment in the other eight counties was put on hold to answer questions advocates raised about accessibility to providers' offices. Opponents of the project in the legislature also called for a slow-down based on anecdotal reports from a few constituents. By the time these issues were cleared up several months later, the entire project was terminated after the two HMOs realized that they were running substantial losses on the contract, primarily because of high prescription drug costs and hospital utilization. Within the year, KP decided first to terminate the entire state contract and then to leave the state (and the Northeast) altogether. Thus, half-way through the project, the coordinator's duties changed from facilitating the transition of care into the HMO and improving HMO-community agency relationships, to facilitating that transition of care *back* to the fee-for-service system.

Despite the upheavals experienced by the project, the coordinator's clear effectiveness led to his hire by KP after demonstration funding for the position ended, even though the original state program transitioning these beneficiaries to managed care programs had also ended. Additional evidence of the coordinator's success was that the state created a similar position to aid the Medicaid/SSI population in the state's Primary Care Case Management System, and they hired the KP coordinator to fill it. Therefore, despite extremely difficult circumstances related to system and legislative changes, the program was remarkably successful in providing and coordinating services for an important at-risk population. Much can be learned from this project so that future efforts can replicate its successes and avoid some of the pitfalls it encountered. Details of the program follow.

Implementation

The demonstration funded the coordinator, who began work on the project the week before the enrollment transitions began. This timing was unfortunate (although unavoidable because of the separate and conflicting state and demonstration timetables), since the coordinator was new to KP and did not know the system well.

To begin work, the coordinator met with all agencies and groups serving individuals under age 65 with physical or mental health disabilities. In addition, he visited all health centers and medical practices in the counties that enrolled SSI/Medicaid members, and provided information and education about the project. The coordinator also worked with a social work intern, who developed a resource manual to be used to aid enrollees. Efforts were modified to effectively target different population groups. For example, the coordinator enlisted the help of Vermont's Independent Living Centers to help train staff in group homes about the project and what it meant for their residents to be in managed care. It became apparent that such training was necessary because many staff did not understand important distinctions among and within systems (e.g., the difference between Medicare and Medicaid).

Beneficiaries were informed of the mandate to enroll in one of the two participating HMOs by an organization experienced in Medicaid enrollment "brokering." Rates of voluntary choice of providers were high—i.e., only about one-fourth were assigned a PCP. Once new members enrolled in KP, they were sent a modified version of the demonstration's HSF, designed to identify the needs of these members. Lists of new Medicaid/SSI enrollees were given to each PCP, and if an HSF was returned, a copy was also sent along. For new members who did not return the HSF, the coordinator arranged to place a blank HSF in the medical record so members could complete it at the time of a their next visit.

The characteristics of the 228 new members who returned HSFs are shown in Table 6.1. Of those returning questionnaires, 48% reported four or more health conditions, and many of these members had hospitalizations in the 12 months before returning the questionnaire (31%); slightly more had ER visits in the prior 6 months (33%). Fewer (13%) needed help with ADLS, but 50% needed help with IADLs. Equipment use was less than in many of the other groups, with only 24% needing some kind of equipment and 3% using a wheelchair. Lastly, only 9% used any of the special treatments assessed in the HSF.

The difficulties in obtaining information through the HSF from this population are reflected in the fact that this represents only a 29% return rate from the 781 individuals who joined KP. This result repeats the experience of the Hawaii NORC project, which had an even lower return rate for health status forms. Even when the form came from the health plan with a letter that said the intended goal was to help serve the new member better, the SSI beneficiaries were reported to be fearful that the information they provided might be used against them in regard to their continued eligibility for benefits. This reaction greatly reduced the utility of this form of information gathering.

The coordinator also played the role of liaison between the state, Vermont Behavioral Health, the Community Rehabilitation and Treatment Program, and the health plan. And, as might have been expected, the work inevitably spilled over into addressing the full range of transition and service issues (e.g., high emergency department use; problems with access to primary care providers in rural areas; members not understanding that they had access to, and should use, primary care providers). With time, the coordinator role encompassed systems coordination, individual care management of SSI/Medicaid members, education of new members about the system and their rightful community care benefits, and across-the-board problem solving—skid greasing, trouble shooting, and crack filling. The complexity of the linkages, the lack of prior coordination between service providers, and the multifaceted nature of the mental and physical health problems and functional limitations of enrollees made individual case management activities a necessary part of the process of linking agencies so that the need for such case management might be reduced in the future.

Provider Feedback

Interviews with project and community agency staff and advocates revealed that coordinating medical and community care may have been easier in the HMO setting than in the fee-for-service environment. The latter environment had no mechanism for supporting coordination of services, whereas funding was available within the HMO. Ironically, advocates for people with disabilities (who had helped to end the managed care program) regretted the loss of the KP coordinator, who had educated beneficiaries about their transportation benefits, helped people maintain their SSI and Medicaid benefits, and helped clarify care-related disputes between agencies.

Additional important lessons were also gleaned from the project. First, the separation of the behavioral health contract from the KP contract was not clean: sometimes it was not clear which organization was the responsible payer (e.g., who should pay for neuropsychiatric assessments—the health plan or the behavioral health care provider?) Second, special needs caused problems in care provision—cognitive impairments led to needs for additional medical services that were not deemed medically necessary (such as increased recovery time in an institutional setting because a member could not take care of himself at home). Stepped-up community care services could resolve such problems, but costs were seen as being shifted to the community agency. In summary, it was difficult to make a clean separation of needs for community care and medical services.

Summary

Working with the SSI/Medicaid population was challenging in a managed care environment, particularly for a health plan relatively new to the political and economic climate of the area in which a project was being implemented. Additionally, care-management needs associated with this population were far more complex than those of Temporary Assistance for Needy Families Medicaid recipients—usually poor mothers and children—who are generally in better health and need far fewer services. SSI/Medicaid members also needed respite care, transportation services, and help maintaining their SSI/Medicaid benefits. However, the distinctions that formal systems made in funding and service delivery were confusing to service users, and often required interpretation and assistance to navigate through them.

As a result of political pressures and Kaiser's financial losses on the program, only 781 persons were enrolled instead of the expected 3,000. This failure might have been prevented if the following had been present: (a) better planning and coordination between the state and health plans, (b) starting with a pilot project to identify problems and methods to address those problems, and (c) having an adequate time commitment (at least two years) from all parties—the state, the legislature, and the health plans—to establish the system. Additionally, the project might have gone more smoothly had the coordinator been available to participate in initial planning processes, and had the systems he created been in place prior to enrolling members. Ultimately, however, even if the enrollment and care coordination processes had been perfect, the inadequacy of the payment rate levels and structures would have still doomed the initiative financially.

Despite these difficulties, the project had many positive outcomes. The time and energy the coordinator devoted to establishing relationships between providers and agencies—to understanding the problems of individual members, to resolving difficulties, and to educating and re-educating providers and agencies—were worthwhile and may have improved care significantly.

The Vermont SSI/Medicaid project provides an excellent example of the multiplicity of services needed by a population of low-income adults with high rates of chronic illness and disability and the problems encountered in coordinating those services. The model was of a linked system of care, with the coordinator often by necessity slipping into a coordination role. Perhaps the needs of the SSI group justified a fully integrated system, where care is provided by an interdisciplinary team managing services across the acute-long-term medical-mental health continuum. This project suggests that linked systems can work, but that the barriers are great. For populations with needs as complex as those served by this project, it is possible that coordinated or even integrated care might lead to better outcomes. Most importantly, this project shows us that even one person in a supported coordinating role can overcome enormous barriers to care between *and* within systems, protecting the most vulnerable individuals.

WHAT WAS LEARNED FROM THE FIVE PROJECTS, TAKEN TOGETHER?

The projects discussed in this chapter identified and characterized additional populations with chronic illnesses and disabilities, and described their needs. They also revealed new constellations of community care services for each population, with their companion issues of access, eligibility, funding, service limitations, and coordination challenges. Specifically, the projects delineated several important issues about identifying and providing services for non-elderly members with disabilities.

First, it was possible to identify a set of members who have great needs for health care services and are at higher risk of mortality than others in the health plan. Administrative records can be used to find these individuals, and, although those who do not apply for disability benefits will be missed using the strategy employed here, a group *can* be identified that needs special care and tailoring of health care to their needs. Further work should expand on this discovery to determine the feasibility of using such information to aid in care provision and preparation for special needs during medical encounters.

Second, the two needs assessment projects indicate that needs for home- and community-based care are great among some groups in the health plan population who are not targeted for community care interventions, for whom linkages to community care are weak, or who do not appear to qualify for community care because their needs are met by informal caregivers, preventing them from being identified or designated as "disabled." The Denver Parents project found that parents of children with disabilities need (a) additional information about their children's' illnesses, (b) information about the availability of support and services, and (c) help linking to those services. Such information and help needs to be offered proactively by health care providers without parents having to push. Additionally, therapy and durable medical equipment benefits may need to be reevaluated for their adequacy.

The Northwest Adults with Disabilities project found that non-elderly adults with relapsing conditions often need ongoing support with house-keeping, meal preparation, transportation, medication administration/management, money management, symptom monitoring, and child care, as well as additional help with these tasks during flare-ups. Such care is not generally provided for, but most of these services could be offered by existing community care programs with minimal changes, particularly if the health plan would facilitate linkages between patients and programs, develop a pre-certification process, and clarify responsibility for payment.

Third, the intervention studies reported here make clear that it is essential to have commitment at the system level that includes a person (or persons) who leads the effort to facilitate system changes and linkages. The three information-only projects discussed in this chapter did not have this change feature, and although they each uncovered and distributed valuable learning about the needs of persons with disabilities, they didn't have the intervention follow-through that seems to be required to make lasting operational changes.

The Vermont SSI/Medicaid effort showed, however, that a systems change strategy may not be enough. When vulnerable populations are involved, case management may also be necessary to coordinate care and information across members, health care providers, the health plan, community care providers, and governmental institutions that fund such care, until links between agencies are well-established. The Vermont SSI/Medicaid project made clear that a coordinator in such a role can make even the worst of situations workable for the most vulnerable members.

Overall, it appears that achieving successful community care programs for children and non-elderly adults will involve several steps. Clearly, reaching out to community agencies to form relationships and exchange information about services provided by each organization must begin the process. Once such relationships are established, there is a need to work out mechanisms for sharing information about referrals and service status to facilitate coordinated care. Medical care providers must be educated about the kinds of services available, the populations served, and appropriate processes of referral to community organizations. When these conditions are met, the health plan should then reach out to members likely to need community services and facilitate connections to those services. Lastly, to be successful in these efforts, there must be support for staff in linkage roles who, in addition to facilitating the above steps in the process, collect, analyze, and report data evaluating the programs and linkages.

7

Situation Analysis:
Challenges and Opportunities,
Strengths and Weaknesses

Walter Leutz, Merwyn Greenlick, and Lucy Nonnenkamp

The United States and many other industrialized countries face both challenges and opportunities over the coming decades in how they address the needs of persons with disabilities and chronic illnesses. If they don't develop, test, and implement system changes, they are likely to find themselves in the worst of both worlds: rising costs for a non-system of services that don't meet the needs of the most vulnerable and expensive groups in society.

One side of the challenge is that rates of disability and chronic illness are rising as the result of population aging and medical interventions that save the lives of younger persons with disabilities. With increasing numbers and diversity of persons with disabilities, the demands for a wide variety of non-medical supports are sure to grow. From the point of view of persons with disabilities and their families, their needs for supportive community care are every bit as important as their needs for medical care interventions that cure illness and prolong life.

The other side of the challenge is that funders continue to feed a medical care system that excludes community care and to starve a community care system that could provide a counterbalance. Medical care systems are becoming ever more specialized, technical, institution-based, and expensive, while systems of community care stagnate, with public funding targeted heavily to limited numbers of the very poor, few requirements for coordination among programs and funding sources, and a near void of public help for the working and middle classes. The two "major" new initiatives for the elderly in the

United States—tax breaks for long-term care insurance and informal care-givers-solidify private and family responsibilities for already-burdened family members.[1]

Ironically, managed care—with a few exceptions—has not proven to be a counter to these patterns, even though managed care has spread among the general population and also has tried to develop special programs for chronic illness and disability. Whereas the rhetoric of the HMO movement historically has been to create population-based programs emphasizing prevention, the last decade's combination of market pressures, payers' cost control efforts, and profit motives have taken the luster off what used to be a movement among committed health care providers to meet the needs of their communities. Now managed care often seems more like a set of techniques for limiting access and controlling utilization. The several managed care efforts to integrate medical and community care/long-term care (e.g., PACE, dual eligible initiatives, Social HMOs, Wisconsin Partnership) are promising concepts, but the multitude of difficulties they face in implementation and scope reveal their limits as vehicles for broader system reform.

With medical costs already high and rising, most people realize the need for limits on spending, but the priorities seem out of balance. Medicare and traditional health insurance are ready to pay for expensive and extensive medical interventions in the hospital for seriously chronically ill and disabled elders, but they won't pay to help the family cope when their loved one is sent home. Systems aren't very good at transitioning from intensive interventions to more supportive care, and even individuals and families and providers who know they should be thinking about quality of life rather than quantity try just one more promising intervention and see life end in the hospital with tubes and monitors and masks rather than at home among family and friends. To paraphrase the popular book about men and women, it often seems like medical care is from Mars and community care is from Venus.

KP's Manifesto 2005 isn't a panacea for transforming and connecting these distant systems, but it offers a vision of how they can approach each other through linking and coordinating mechanisms. It acknowledges the challenges in the demographic and health care environments, but it also sees opportunities.

The Manifesto's first premise is that medical care needs to acknowledge the importance of the functional limitations of disability and the services that address those needs. A corollary is that only by engaging those needs and services can medical care begin to see how other kinds of help can fit and to understand the importance of these kinds of help to patients.

---

[1] Although are a few countervailing examples to these trends, this is the general direction of development in the United State in particular.

Its second premise is that formal care systems should be building on the strengths and preferences of persons with disabilities and their families rather than just trying to shore up their weaknesses. Persons with disabilities and their families and other advocates have built the movement for deinstitutionalization and community care, and, primarily through the family, they continue to provide the bulk of the care delivered. Systems that empower people to do what they want and get what they want may find that people not only want something different than what formal care would have offered, they often want less. Professionals, especially in medical care, would do well to begin to listen more closely to these preferences.

A third premise is that medical care should be trying to help identify and access community support and services for its patients. Concurrently, it should be trying to build bridges for communication and cooperation with community care agencies. A corollary here is that there is something worth finding on the other side of those bridges, and that patients will be well served.

Its fourth premise is that appropriate kinds of care should move from institutions to community settings, particularly the home. Obviously, this does not mean that the hospital or even the doctor's office should go away, but rather that there is an opportunity to takes steps towards building community-based, public-health-oriented systems of care (Andersen & Pourat, 1997).

A final premise behind the Manifesto is that the politics of medical care and community care can be changed for the better. The only thing that people consistently like in the U.S. health care system is their doctor. Larger system characteristics—coverage, cost, and access—are widely disliked, as is managed care itself. The Manifesto posits that redirecting medical care and community care toward a community-based public health model could revive the public's involvement and investment in both systems. Since community care is so much a matter of state and local policy and programming, and since the Manifesto's model addresses the needs of all persons with disabilities, it may provide the basis to build practical political support.

This brief review of challenges and opportunities in the environment borrows from the framework of strategic planning, and that framework is followed through these last two chapters. Next assessed are the capacities of KP and the community organizations it worked with to carry out the Manifesto's vision. What strengths and weaknesses were identified? Were members with disabilities and their family members included and in agreement with these visions? The chapter ends by setting some broad strategic goals and reviewing why it is worthwhile to move in this direction. These lessons are drawn from the KP demonstration experience, but they are relevant to other coordinated health care systems.

The next chapter draws on lessons learned about creating a linkage and coordination system to sketch a "mature" system for better connecting medical and community care. It concludes with some recommendations for creating such a system and some reflections on overall prospects.

SYSTEM STRENGTHS AND WEAKNESSES IDENTIFIED IN THE DEMONSTRATION

The general premise of Manifesto 2005 is that the medical care and community care systems can be taken pretty much as they are and adjusted to work more closely together for the benefit of individuals with disabilities. To assess the feasibility of this notion, review is made of what the demonstration revealed about the strengths and weaknesses of the two systems, both in terms of providing their own services and in terms of their current levels of cooperation. Also assessed are learnings about persons with disabilities and their families concerning their needs, use, and preferences concerning assistance. The points to be made are summarized in Box 7.1.

Medical Care

It was not the purpose of the demonstration to either describe or evaluate the overall quality or delivery of medical care to KP members with disabilities. There were some apparent ways that medical care could be improved that were identified in proposals that were rejected, but the review team was not able to support or pursue them. Instead, the demonstration mostly supported projects around the edges of medical care. But in the process of developing these projects, some things were learned about how the medical system works for persons with disabilities.

First, since KP offers medical care as an entitlement to members, formal access to covered medical care services was not a problem. KP members by definition had coverage for a defined package of core medical benefits. Physicians used diagnoses to help assess their need for additional services, including hospitals, nursing facility rehabilitation, and home health. In contrast to what was found in community care, there were no additional eligibility or financial barriers within the entitled system of care other than relatively trivial copays for some services.

Second, there were some practical barriers to access, however, as well as some service delivery practices that seemed to get in the way of good care. Standard office visits were at times too short and lacked needed supports for persons with disabilities. Project staff reported that the complexity of chronic illnesses, disability-related issues such as transfers, cognitive deficits, and the

---

BOX 7.1   Demonstration Lessons about Medical Care, Community Care, and Persons with Disabilities and their Caregivers

---

Medical Care System
- Relative to the numerous barriers to community care, medical care provides easy access to covered services based on doctors' orders.
- For the most disabled, standard office visits may be too short and lack needed supports.
- Outpatient medical providers are not experienced in the management of complex "care-in-place" needs of dependent and vulnerable members.
- Physicians don't talk to their patients much about functional status, overall personal goals, caregiving, or community care.
- Physicians often are reluctant to change but will ask and refer in clear-cut cases.
- Other medical care staff are concerned with functioning and can lead linkage efforts.
- Medical care staff need expanded job descriptions and time to connect with community care.
- Community care referrals, follow-up, and monitoring are hampered by information system gaps.
- Disability predicts high medical costs, but members with disabilities are not easily identified in medical information systems.
- Home care benefit expansions can serve unmet needs at low cost.

Community Care System
- Resources were found and connections established in every community.
- Core service constellations varied by group (e.g., elders used personal care, homemaker, day care, transportation, respite).
- General models are needed, but in the end, all linkage is local.
- Personal relationships are key.
- Community care providers are eager but cautious partners.
- There are barriers to community care services, e.g., cost, applications, transportation, location, wait lists.
- It is easier to establish linkage than coordination.

Service Users and Caregivers
- Users and caregivers should be a part of planning.
- Disability and service needs are showcased by linkage projects.
- People appreciate medical care's efforts at linkage.
- Family caregivers are the major system resource, and they have needs too.
- Individuals with disabilities are diverse in terms of class, living arrangements, needs, preferences, types of disabilities, age, gender, race, and more.
- Formal systems can disempower service users and also empower them through better information, smoother access, building on users' strengths, and developing the care plan around the user's goals.
- Self-help organizations and groups provide unique connections and support.
- What people want may be less than and different from what providers think.

participation of caregivers required extra time that was not available in the standard visit. Another related shortcoming was the heavy reliance on family caregivers to help with compliance, monitoring, transportation, and other logistics, and the lack of a back-up system if the caregiver was weak or absent.

These issues converged for foster home residents, who often lacked both transportation and an involved caregiver who could accompany them to appointments to give and receive information about symptoms and care. The lack of supports may have been behind this group's abnormally low rates of clinic visits and prevention procedures and abnormally high use of emergency rooms and hospitals.

Third, primary care physicians and other outpatient medical staff were not experienced in developing, implementing, and monitoring complex medical regimens for their patients in the home and other community-based settings. Such "care-in-place" practice could be a key to maintaining stability for patients with complex chronic illnesses and in turn reducing emergency department visits and hospital stays. It would also support families in their struggles to oversee complex medical and skilled care regimens.

Fourth, similar to the studies of fee-for-service physicians reviewed in Chapter 1, project after project showed that KP physicians did not consistently engage their frail patients in conversations about such things as functional status, community care needs, community care services, or caregiver issues. For example, pre-implementation focus groups of family caregivers for dementia patients reported that primary care physicians and neurologists had not made an early diagnosis or had not provided information about community resources or about the progress of disease. Focus groups of parents of children with disabilities found similar shortfalls.

The many projects that tried to educate and train physicians to identify and refer their particular patient group were generally disappointed with results. Project staff reached out to physicians in grand rounds and individual and team meetings. They gave out brochures, prescription pads, and the like. At most sites, few referrals resulted. Project staff seldom expressed surprise at this, however, because they understood how busy physicians were and how many other demands they faced. Perhaps changing physician practice behavior take more time than the demonstration allowed. Staff were confident that behavior would change over the long run, as linkage mechanisms improved and services became better understood. But staff still felt the short-run irony that a referral by a physician was one of the strongest aids to getting a patient to try a service.[2]

---

[2] Based on this experience, getting physicians to attend regular team meetings around patients—as envisioned in the full integration model—would be next to impossible without the resources to buy out their clinic times.

Fifth, in contrast to the difficulties most projects had in enlisting physicians' active support, there were several bright spots with physicians' participation. The brightest were neurologists in the dementia project. When asked
why they hesitated to diagnose dementia, physicians replied that they hated
giving families such devastating news and not having anything to offer. After
implementation of the post-diagnosis protocol, diagnosis rates rose, as did
referrals to the single point of contact. Neurologists were pleased to report
that they had "discovered" that they could offer help with caregiver support,
advance directives, and financial planning. On the other end of the age scale,
similar results were achieved with pediatricians, who, after receiving training
in what early intervention and other special needs agencies could do, and
with support of a new team structure, increased their rates of direct referrals.
These two projects showed that physicians will become involved when the
project addresses a problem they encounter and offers information and system supports that are responsive and relatively clear.

Sixth, in contrast to primary care physicians' near singular focus on medical care issues, the demonstration stimulated proposals from a wide range of
other medical professionals who were interested in functioning, informal
caregiving, and community care services. These were the discharge planners,
clinic social workers, continuing care (home health) nurses, and specialty
clinic staff (e.g., geriatrics, special needs kids, diabetes, dementia). These staff
knew about and worried about the shortcomings in care after medical home
care benefits expired. By empowering these individuals with funds and status, the demonstration raised their prominence and the importance of issues
of disability and community care.

Seventh, without this explicit and material support, these potential community care leaders would not have been empowered. Their proposals also
showed that in the absence of a special effort like the demonstration, even
such a relatively well-organized and well-staffed HMO as KP lacked basic
linkage and coordination mechanisms. Social work and nursing staff had
concerns about how well frail members were being cared for in the community, but they did not have what they needed to act on those concerns. One
problem was that prior to the demonstration, they did not have the time to
acquire first-hand knowledge of community care system, agencies, or staff.
In part because of this lack of familiarity, providers reported hesitancy to
make community care referrals. Another barrier to making referrals was fear
that patients would return from community care referrals with complaints
about service adequacy, relevance, accessibility, or cost. Lacking first-hand,
personal contact with community care agencies and staff, the typical medical
care referral to community care put all the onus for making the connection
on patients and families.

The project staff addressed these gaps in connections by simply getting
out into the community to talk to the agencies they wanted to connect to.

Their mere presence was important since it showed that KP cared about community care services; and in the visits staff gathered up-to-date eligibility, fee and contact information, and also brought back brochures and even community agency staff to do training. Health plan staff served on community boards and committees. They set up simple but effective ways to make referrals work better. For example, in the post-diagnosis dementia protocol developed with the Alzheimer's Association (AA), there was a provision for KP to to get the member to sign a release, which was faxed to the AA and thereby allowed the AA to call. These connections are discussed in the next section.

Eighth, another barrier to turning the system's focus to disability and community care services was that medical records and information systems lacked these kinds of data. In contrast, medical system diagnoses, treatments, encounters, and referrals appeared in the KP electronic medical record for all providers to see. This allowed providers in any location to follow up and inquire about current status of a service or treatment. Without similar fields in the record for functional status and community care referrals, providers and care managers didn't know what to inquire about.

With the exception of the adult foster home project and one adult day project at the Group Health site in Seattle, demonstration efforts to change the medical record were unsuccessful, but the next chapter shows that useful models were proposed. The utility of having this kind of information was illustrated in the project to try to identify members with disabilities through HMO medical and administrative records. Although the project was not able to identify data sources that would confirm current disability or identify new disability, the project showed that members who had asked for documentation for disability claims had extremely high utilization years after their applications. Having accurate information on disability would be a powerful way to identify at risk members.

Finally, one other demonstration medical system initiative in community care deserves mention: pilot expansions of home care benefits that were tied in closely to covered home health and continuing care teams. The two projects that tested such expansions found that continuing care could identify patients who (largely because of weak family supports) needed care even though they didn't qualify for skilled home health care, or who needed more than home health would cover. One site targeted post-acute patients, while the other targeted dementia patients. Rather than partnering with community home care agencies, both sites chose to place the home care aides in the KP continuing care team and to manage and pay for the services themselves. The post-acute aides provided primarily personal care and housekeeping, but for surprisingly short periods, while the dementia aides helped primarily with IADLs, including paperwork, making appointments, and accompanying members to medical care visits. Questions for future investigation are who should pay for such service extensions and whether in a better developed system it would make more sense to keep them within the medical care system or to place them in a community agency.

Community Care

The central hypotheses of the demonstration were (a) that there would be valuable resources in the community for persons with disabilities and their caregivers, and (b) that it would be possible for the medical care system to strengthen connections to those resources. How did the projects support or refute these hypotheses?

First, projects were able to find community care resources in every demonstration community, and it was generally possible to improve member and health system connections to them. Most of the sites worked with only a single type of service, but putting all the sites together shows the wide range of services and agencies that deliver community care. Sites tapped into volunteer organizations such as churches, advocacy/service organizations like the Alzheimer's Association (both local and national branches) and the Rosyln Carter Center for caregiving, a wide range of providers (adult day services, personal care and homemaker agencies, transportation services, adult foster care), and care management agencies (from early intervention for babies and their families to the aging network for elders). Most of the service agencies were small and independent rather than parts of large chains, although most also had national trade or advocacy arms with more capabilities.

Second, by including projects that addressed the needs of persons with disabilities other than elders, the demonstration showed that distinct constellations of agencies, finances, and services are related to each of the several categories of individuals with disabilities (e.g., newborns, school-age children, adults with physical disabilities, adults with intellectual disabilities, elders, SSI eligibles). Doing an effective job connecting with community care for all persons with disabilities will require reconnaissance about how to access these separate systems, how service users and families experience them, and what the linkage issues are.

Third, while each group (e.g., elders) had a core set of community services and funding sources that should be considered in a core "package" to link to, Tip O'Neill's comment about the nature of politics can be paraphrased to apply: "All linkage is local." General types of agencies and funding could be looked to for help with particular types of disabilities, but the specifics were different in each local project. For example, adult day services regulations differed in Oregon, California, and Washington, and this was associated with different capabilities of agencies and different financing available for participants. Joint protocols that were developed across regions had to be tailored to local opportunities and barriers. And there were differences within the medical system too, which meant, for example, that different units within KP led the same multi-site project locally.

Fourth, a key component of successful linkage projects was the personal relationships that were developed across the systems. The only way to have such relationships was to work on developing and maintaining them by visiting community agencies and having them come to KP to do training, by attending community network meetings, and by serving on agency boards. When KP staff turned up at places that medical staff were seldom seen, they were noticed.

Fifth, community agencies were eager yet cautious about working with KP to develop connections. The eager side related to the chances for increased referrals, improving care, and even tapping into KP funds. The caution stemmed from suspicions that KP might try to use community services in order to save on medical care. Demonstration sites were more successful when they fulfilled these hopes and were sensitive to the sources of caution. Most did indeed increase referrals and also produced better referrals. A few sites followed the "law" that "integration costs before it pays" and purchased services from community care agencies (e.g., contracting for volunteer recruitment and management, paying educators to lead caregiving classes). Another bonus for both sides was the positive publicity each side got from associating with the other.

An example of this arose soon after the demonstration, when KP California was sued by a disability special interest group because the limited design of some facilities was a barrier to people with disabilities. One of the physician leaders of the project seeking to identify members with disabilities through application records for disability insurance shared a copy of overheads from a project presentation as a case-in-point of KP's interest in improving care for members with disabilities. The information seemed to improve KP's image with the plaintiffs, and the settlement included significant commitments to upgrade facilities regarding accessibility to person with physical mobility limitations.

There was no evidence that KP tried to use community services to do its job, and the closer connection with community agencies seemed to help agencies to understand that. For example, the community managers of early intervention services said that having a clear "no" from KP about covering a particular service helped them to access other sources of funds to pay for services. The explicit negative response was better than not being able to get a straight answer.

Sixth, lest the picture of community care get artificially bright, there were many shortfalls in community care services and in members' access to them. Since community care is typically provided by small and independent agencies supported by different funding, members faced a variety of application processes that screened on the basis of disability level, income, geography, and other factors. Lack of funds to pay and waiting lists for publicly funded services were often barriers to personal care, transportation, and adult day services for elders. Transportation and location were also barriers to using community-based services such as day care and the classes offered in the demonstration's caregiver workshops. Lack of respite care was an additional barrier to the latter. Besides access barriers, there was some evidence of quality and reliability problems. Community care providers used primarily paraprofessional staff, sometimes with some nursing support. Staff turnover, limited training, and lack of supervision were identified as problems in some settings (e.g., foster care, personal care aides). These problems might have been worse had the demonstration not been conducted primarily in states with above-average public service coverage and care coordination, at least for low-income elders: California, Oregon, Washington, Colorado, and Hawaii.

Seventh, mirroring the medical care side, the community care agencies did not have much linkage infrastructure or activity prior to the demonstration initiatives. In developing connections, the demonstration sites included mostly "linkage" projects but also a few that sought closer collaboration through "coordination." The linkage projects typically did two things. First, they tried to help KP learn about a particular community care service, who should use it, and how to apply. This was done through sharing brochures, bringing in community care staff for in-service training, and so on. Second, they tried to set up referral and communication systems to tell the community agency when potential clients were coming over from medical care, to give feedback to KP about whether they got there, and then to talk back and forth about ongoing issues. The first part of this infrastructure was easier to establish than the second part, particularly because of the difficulty getting community care information into medical information systems. In practice, most sites used a "manual" system in the person of a designated single point of contact within the medical system to handle the information and follow-up.

"Coordination," which builds case management and clinical cooperation on top of the linkage system, was more difficult to establish. Coordination seeks to get medical care and community care providers working to support each other in the care of patients who may need the most complex care in both systems. An example would be medical care's learning that a patient was receiving personal care assistance from a particular agency and providing the agency with information about diet, prescriptions, and symptoms to watch for. In turn, community care would support prescribed diet and medication regimens and appropriate medical providers about suspicious symptoms or behavior. With the exception of some adult day centers and adult foster homes (discussed presently), community care providers did not have staff or supervisors who were trained to do this or the systems to help staff coordinate in these ways. Moreover, these agencies reported that they lacked standing with medical care to either receive or convey these types of information.

The adult day care projects tried to take on some of these coordination roles, but they were were frustrated by the lack of a reliable link for the information needed for coordination. Perhaps part of the problem was the projects' failure to greatly increase the use of day care, which would have justified more investment in health plan systems. Although adult day care referrals and usage increased marginally at all sites, there was resistance to the service both among members (costs, leaving home, other people) and medical providers (member resistance, not knowing whom to refer).

In contrast to the day care sites, the foster care providers were already serving large numbers of KP members, and the providers were responsible for day-to-day care. However, the foster homes' small size, their providers' limited training, and their tight staffing left them without the capacity to take on a truly interactive relationship. On the medical side, the project's attempt to set up case management across system boundaries was unable to provide needed support to outpatient medical visits, to track foster care discharges and admissions (other than from a hospital), or to find a way to improve communications about prescription drug changes and monitoring. Also, even if the foster care providers were more knowledgeable and available, it was not clear that KP primary care physicians and outpatient care staff had the "care-in-place" systems to support them from office-based practice. The long-term care program's pilot that sends members of physician/nurse practitioner teams to adult foster homes is an attempt to put into place a system to support an adult foster home "care-in-place" system.

Members and Families

In one sense, it feels odd to include individuals with disabilities and their families in an assessment of strengths and weaknesses. They are the ones that the system is supposed to be serving. But in another sense, they are at the heart of the system in terms of the amount of care that is provided and of how their preferences, and even personal strengths and weaknesses, affect how they use, don't use, and otherwise shape the formal system.

This section summarizes and reflects on what was learned in the demonstration about people with disabilities and their family caregivers. Like the summaries of learning about the medical care and community care, the synthesis draws from disparate projects that weren't designed to sum up to the whole. Particularly in the case of people with disabilities, the emphasis was on finding individuals who would use particular services rather than on characterizing distinct populations of people with disabilities (e.g., elders, special needs children) within the larger population of members. This limits what can be said about projecting findings across projects or into the larger population of members.

Another limitation—and this is also the first lesson—is that few of the demonstration's service projects involved people with disabilities in their design and implementation. Because there was no requirement for such involvement in the basic demonstration design, this is the fault of designers much more than that of the project leaders. The completed projects give insights into people with disabilities and families from their responses to the baseline HSF, from satisfaction surveys and interviews performed by some projects, and from their use of project services. A few other projects used focus groups to learn about the problems and desires of potential service users. And others involved advocacy groups. All in all, there is a story to tell, but it would have been a much richer and more useful story if there had been more efforts to involve people with disabilities and their caregivers in planning, implementation, and evaluation. Next time.

The second lesson is that chronic illness and disability exist in health care systems, and that they imply needs for help beyond medical care. This was no surprise to anyone, but these projects that were designed to reach out to particular populations of people with disabilities lent reality to the abstract statistics. They identified significant numbers of members using or needing services such as adult day care, personal care, transportation, foster care, early intervention, caregiver training and support, and extra help for temporary disability. Project staff believed that even more members could have been identified and referred with more effective and aggressive systems that include, for example, more consistent physician referrals and screening of administrative and clinical databases.

The third lesson is that (despite lack of user involvement at the ground level) linkage and coordination were issues that resonated with people with disabilities and their caregivers. Members responded to outreach and referral initiatives concerning the projects, and they appreciated that their health plan was taking an interest. Most projects served elders, but other groups using concurrent medical care and community care services due to disability were easily identified and involved (e.g., parents of infants and school-age children, working-age adults). The community care agencies and medical care specialties they used differed by group, but they all had issues both about the responsiveness and adequacy of core medical care and community care services, as well as linkage between the two systems.

The fourth lesson is that caregivers were everywhere and did everything. They were the primary allies of both medical care and community care in providing direct help to people with disabilities and in managing logistics and communication for each system and between the two systems. Individuals with serious disabilities who lacked caregivers faced the greatest difficulties obtaining adequate community care and medical care in the community. But the projects—particularly the caregiver training project—showed that caregivers differed in their capabilities and their life cycle status. Relationships to the caregiver and the outside world were factors in completion of the workshops and in gaining competence. The workshops also confirmed that caregivers were themselves at risk: Being too busy with caregiving was a major reason for not even starting classes. The different patterns of not taking and not completing the courses sent a message to the project leaders that follow-up outreach had to be organized to support some of the most needy and vulnerable caregivers. Different levels, types, and amounts of support needs to be available to meet the varying needs of caregivers.

Fifth, the diversity of members with disabilities was remarkable. They differed in their financial resources and their willingness to spend resources on services. They differed in their preferences for particular services (e.g., some loved adult day care but most didn't) and for using formal help at all. A project that tried to organize services for residents of elderly high-rise condominiums found that residents who were not part of KP were suspicious of health plan staff and mostly wanted to be left alone.

A sixth lesson is that formal systems were often seen as alien and disempowering. Frustrations with community care started with obtaining useful information about what was available, continued with the need to go through extensive application and screening processes, and were compounded by having to do it all over again for each separate service. Priorities defined over and over again in focus groups and interviews included good information, ease of entry, and being treated with respect. A key ingredient in respect was for professionals and program designs to focus on the strengths/positive sides of people with disabilities and caregivers rather than just seeing problems and offering solutions.

This last point leads to a seventh lesson: self-help groups and advocacy organizations were an invaluable resource. Through the Alzheimer's Association, for example, the demonstration tapped into both national expertise and local networks of formal services and volunteer support. Dementia caregivers made quick and strong connections to others who had been through the experience and who could offer first-hand insights into the course of the illness, the best local services, and how to prepare for finances and decision-making. Similarly, caregiver support groups sprung up spontaneously in the caregiver training project, and they figured in other projects as well. They were not what everyone wanted, but they were just what some people needed.

The eighth and final lesson is that a little goes a long way in helping with community care. None of the demonstration projects was overwhelmed with demands that they did not feel they could meet—either in terms of the numbers of members who sought help (demand was usually less than anticipated) or of how much help people wanted from community care. Although there were certainly individuals who needed more than they could afford or than the system would offer them, the more frequent gap was that the user's or family's priorities did not match the system's service offerings. People wanted help when and where they needed it. Respite care and easy-to-use transportation/escort services were good examples of services that were difficult to arrange to meet actual needs. Volunteers were sometimes the perfect fit in these circumstances.

GOALS

Based on these lessons from the demonstration, a series of goals for the system as a whole, for medical care, and for community care are discussed below and summarized in Box 7.2.

Strategic Goals

The overall strategic goal is to create community-based, public health support systems for people with disabilities. In such a system, an emphasis on prevention and health promotion is supplemented by a strong system of supportive services. An infrastructure for cooperative information, communication, and care management helps clinicians make decisions based on multiple perspectives (Greenlick, 1992). Medical care and community care providers cooperate in sharing information and planning care according to the needs and desires of service users.

A supporting strategic goal is to empower people with disabilities and caregivers to help design and monitor the system and to choose how they will be helped. To date, effective participation has been more common in programs for children with disabilities and persons with intellectual disabilities, and models could be borrowed from there. Bringing advocates and consumers into the planning and policy process will not only add the value of their perspectives, but will also ensure that everyone understands challenges and constraints.

A third strategic goal is to add resources to community care. The community care system will never be able to fulfill its end of the linkage/coordination bargain without substantial improvements in the quantity and quality of its services. Rather than despair about how far there is to go, advocates should consider recent decades' increases in funding as momentum to be promoted through continuing improvements in results.

These strategic goals could be pursued by a single health care system such as KP working with its local community, or they could be pursued by communities as a whole—that is, all medical care and community care providers

---

BOX 7.2   Goals for System Reform

Strategic Goals

- Create community-based, public health support systems for persons with disabilities.
- Empower persons with disabilities and caregivers to help design and monitor the system and to choose how they will be helped.
- Add resources to community care and redirect balance of spending on persons with disabilities toward community care.

Medical System Goals

- Empower linkage professionals to raise consciousness of functional status and assistance, create and maintain community care connections, and manage single points of contact.
- Design a way for members, families, and community caregivers to directly deposit new symptoms and information of concern to the single point of contact.
- Reach out to persons with disabilities and their caregivers through screening, targeted referral points, multi-faceted communications, and just-in-time screening of databases.
- Include physicians on a "needs to know" and "needs to tell" basis.
- Expand the medical record to include functional status and community care information.
- Review and clarify benefit limits and consider modest extensions to bridge gaps.

Community Care Goals

- Clarify constellations of services and financing for distinct groups of persons with disabilities.
- Create assessment and care planning systems that build on strengths and empower service users.
- Create single points of entry for all regardless of income.
- Participate in linkage activities (training about services, referral communications) and (for some) coordination activities (two-way care planning and support).
- Find and use new funds to fix local shortcomings (e.g., fill gaps, reduce waits, improve training and wages).

---

and citizens working on behalf of the whole community. More specific structures and steps to make this happen will be discussed in the next chapter.

Medical Care Goals

The goals proposed for medical care are on a more practical level than the strategic goals. The first step is to designate and empower individuals and groups within medical care systems who can lead the change process. Most of these leaders will not be physicians, although the political commitment of physicians and administrators will be critical. The job of these change agents is to put a consciousness of disability, caregiving, and community care options on the map in medical care systems, to establish connections with community care resources, and to create systems to manage the flow of information and individual service users back and forth across the two systems.

The second goal is to create a way for members, families, and other community caregivers to easily share new symptoms and information of concern to the SPOC. Ideally this would not just be another avenue to get advice from medical care providers to "come to the office so I can see it," but rather a place to get advice and dialogue. Also, the information should have the status to find its way into the medical record for other providers to see and use.

The third goal is for medical care to make systematic connections with its patients with chronic illnesses and disabilities. This includes reviewing and augmenting established population screening systems (e.g., KP was way ahead of the screening requirements added to Medicare managed care in 1997), working with staff at key transition points to identify and refer at risk patients, and also communicating directly with people with disabilities and caregivers through mass media, tailored brochures, and individualized outreach. Medical care needs to be prepared for the predictable events of common syndromes and be ready to respond to this just-in-time sharing of information with care-in-place as an alternative to the "medical cure" intervention model.

The fourth goal is to involve physicians in a realistic and effective manner. The demonstration confirmed the current difficulty of and obstacles to getting physicians to attend to all the details of functioning, caregiving, and community care services. But also showed that physicians will steer patients towards help that they understand and value, especially if there is a team to support them. The trick is to get physicians the information they need to know in order to get them to enter a dialog with patients that leads to an appropriate referral—most likely to the single point of contact.

The involvement of physicians and other clinicians in linkage and coordination would be furthered by action on a fourth goal: to expand the medical record to include information about functional status, caregiving, and community care. In an automated system such as much of KP, this would take the form of a pop-out on the medical record desktop that would advise clinicians of the last known status of key items and prompt them to ask, update, and act as necessary. Another enhancement would be to use the existing clues from automated databases to implement a disability alert when a member requests medical release to apply for disability, or is discharged from the hospital to residential assisted living or group homes.

The fifth and final goal for medical care is to review the limits of current benefits that border community care and to consider clarifications and revisions. The key question is how do service users experience the movements across borders: Are there confusions that could be clarified about what's covered and what's not? Are there modest gaps that could be filled? Key areas are home care services on the borders of skilled home health, transportation, and durable medical equipment and devices.

Community Care Goals

It is more difficult to propose goals for community care than for medical care. In part this is because Manifesto 2005 originated in an organized medical care system, which had the coherence and the resources to initiate action. Even beyond KP, it is the responsibility of medical care to make the first moves toward linkage, coordination, and the ultimate creation of a community-based public health model of care. Community care does not have the resources, the standing, or the leverage to move medical care in this direction. Thus the goals proposed for community care concerning better medical care connections assume substantial responsibility on the medical care side. Nevertheless, most of the community care goals that would enhance linkage with medical care are worth pursuing in themselves.

The first goal is to clarify the services and procedures of community care systems for new service users and for professionals outside these systems who try to work with them. The demonstration showed that there are constellations of services and financing for distinct categories of persons with disabilities. These constellations may be clear to insiders working with each population group, but they are confusing and frustrating for people who are just entering the system. Clear written material and easy connections to help lines, preferably including experienced users, would be a good start.

The second goal is to have assessment and care planning approaches that empower service users. Rather than just collecting information on illness and deficits and dependence and then offering the service that's available as the solution, the focus of assessment should move towards understanding the service user's definition of problems and needs, capitalizing on the strengths of service users and caregivers, and trying to honor preferences with flexible service responses.

The third goal is to create single points of entry into the service constellations appropriate to specific populations. These entry points would be well publicized, easy to contact, have good information, help people understand their service and financing options, and connect people to the types and levels of assistance they may need. Many if not most people with moderate needs and good self-direction could manage on their own with some self-assessment and service option information from the contact point. Others with more complex needs will need more help. This kind of information and triage help should be available to all regardless of income level. Many states and localities already do this for some groups, but much more could be done.

Fourth, community care organizations should do what they can to participate in linkage and coordination activities with medical care. Community care weaknesses in many locales (e.g., lack of coordination, weak staff training and supervision, limited public funding) will hamper more sophisticated forms of coordination, but most of the linkage initiatives tried in the demonstration (helping medical care understand services, referral communications) are feasible. Established relationships will create "standing" for community care providers and service coordinators when they try to give or obtain information from medical care. Analogous to the medical system's reliance on family members for information about symptoms and behavior or to help with compliance, medical care could come to rely on community care providers in situations where the family is weak or absent. Instead of calling 911, formal caregivers could call the medical care single point of contact, or other type of help line, as a first alternative in non-emergencies.

Finally, somehow, somewhere, community care must find additional funding to fix the variety of weaknesses that exist in every community-at least in the United States. These vary somewhat from state to state and community to community, so documenting the need for funds and trying to find them is another piece of the rationale for community planning and development.

CONCLUSION: WHY LINK?

To close this chapter, it is useful to reconsider the question of why a health care plan—or why health care policy makers—should consider going to the bother of creating community care linkages along the lines being discussed, and why community care should cooperate. The simple reason is that there are benefits to service users, health care providers, and medical and community care systems. Some of these benefits are immediate and limited, but progress and advantages can be cumulative and synergistic in support of major system transformation. The reasons to improve linkage and coordination are discussed below and summarized in Box 7.3.

Access

The first reason to more closely connect medical care and community care is to improve access to both community care and medical care services for people who are among the most frequent and complex users of both systems. Patients with disabilities turn up in medical settings; they have needs for community care supports (even if they don't always feel comfortable in

---

**BOX 7.3　Why Link and Coordinate Community Care
and Medical Care?**

Access

- People get more community care and they get it more easily.
- Medical care visits are more productive and meet the needs of patients and caregivers.

Effectiveness and quality

- Better compliance and communication can improve health outcomes.
- Capabilities of community care providers are expanded.
- Reducing caregiver stress may cut mortality and morbidity.

Efficiency

- Management of borders reduces duplication.
- Empowered service users manage their own care.

User empowerment and choice

- Newly disabled get the information and support they need to use complex systems.
- Many can manage on their own, but sometimes more help is needed to understand options and reach goals.

Staff satisfaction and job enhancement

- New options and connections give peace of mind and more power.

Public image and support

- Linkage initiatives counter negative images of medical care and community care systems.

System transformation

- Changing consciousness of community care needs and solutions is a prelude to change in medical care practices.
- Increasing reliance on community care is a path to strengthening it.

---

bringing them up); and the medical system can do something to help them get more community care more easily. In turn, better community care supports can improve access to medical care services by providing support to make and keep appointments, transportation to medical offices, and companion services to make visits more productive.

Effectiveness and Quality

Besides improving access, there are a number of ways linkage—and especially coordination—can enhance the quality and effectiveness of both medical care and community care and yield better health outcomes. What goes on in the home affects the need for and success of medical care. Medical care providers rely on well-informed patients and family caregivers to see that medications are taken as ordered, to monitor status in relation to such conditions as CHF and diabetes, to follow nutrition and hydration needs, and to communicate about symptoms. When informal caregivers are weak or absent, formal community care providers can serve these functions if they can coordinate with medical care. The ability to operate on this plane also improves the quality and effectiveness of community care. The health of family caregivers is a concomitant concern, given the associations between burden and mortality and morbidity. Timely and effective relief of burden through better information, smooth care coordination, and direct community care services may have important health outcome offsets.

Efficiency

Closer coordination of medical care and community care can yield utilization and cost offsets for both medical care and community care. These offsets were not proven in the demonstration, but they were glimpsed. A first-order source of efficiency is from clarifying and coordinating overlapping coverage and services in the community. By clarifying where one system leaves off and the other begins, a coordinated system not only helps people access services across borders, it can also reduce duplication. For example, a coordinated system can avoid sending in skilled home health aides and paraprofessional home care to do the same jobs for the same people. A linked system might be able to avoid some calls to 911 and subsequent emergency room visits if an accessible help line were available. There was a promising reduction in hospital stays for patients without informal caregivers in the project that provided short-term aides for patients with temporary functional declines. There is also efficiency in community care to be realized through better informed and more empowered service users and informal caregivers. They will be more often able to make their own choices and manage their own care.

User Empowerment and Choice

Linkage and coordination foster empowerment and choice for service users by facilitating their use of complex, confusing, and intimidating systems of care. There's something flawed about the notion of pure autonomy for individuals with functional limitations, low incomes, and burdened caregivers facing off against such systems. The linkage and coordination model is based on the idea of "contextual autonomy" (Capitman & Sciegaj, 1995), which acknowledges the limitations on choice in a particular situation and then helps service users make informed choices and achieve goals to the extent possible. Medical care providers are uniquely well-positioned to help newly disabled individuals and their families understand their situations and their community care options, and to aid them in connecting with help. From there, many people with disabilities desire and are able to manage their own care needs, and for many others, families provide all that is needed in direct care and management. However, the need for more active linkage and coordination continues for service users who are most at risk in terms of complexity of medical and functional support needs and fragility of informal support systems.

Staff Satisfaction and Job Enhancement

Having better connections to community care seemed to have intrinsic value for medical care staff who were concerned about what was happening in the community to their most vulnerable patients. Rationales for many of the projects included fears about sending patients home after hospitalizations without enough home health services and with weak family support, or about cutting off home health too early. In the demonstration, staff worries about discharging frail but non-skilled patients were eased by the small extensions of skilled home health afforded by the home health aide in the temporary decline project. Similarly, the community health worker's help with compliance, access, and home-based information gave the continuing care staff a stronger system for helping dementia patients and their caregivers. Effective linkage and coordination can expand the power of medical care staff to do a better job and, in turn, improve their satisfaction with their work. Parallel improvements on the community care side can be hypothesized.

Public Image and Support

By promoting linkage and coordination, medical care and community care systems can counter some of their negative public images. As managed care in its various forms has spread across the United States, the entire medical care system has become infected. The reaction to managed care is not so much against management per se, but rather against the perception that managed care organizations are depriving their members of needed services. The KP Manifesto 2005 concept is just the opposite. The initiative shows that there can still be "care" in managed care, and not just for so-called "healthy" members. Perhaps the most dramatic example were the dementia project's focus groups. They showed that prior to the project, caregivers for dementia patients were surprised and disappointed that their doctors and HMO did not provide much help. After the implementation, the testimonies from members reflected gratitude to see KP helping. This was the pattern in virtually all projects.

System Transformation

The ultimate reason for caring about connecting medical care and community care is that it may be a key ingredient for transforming the way care systems deal with chronic illness and disability. Rather than deal in separate systems—one too medicalized, institutionalized, and expensive and the other fragmented and under-funded—there is an opportunity to create a more community-oriented, coordinated, and stronger system. Practicing in systems with new options will keep medical care current and relevant to changing approaches to chronic illness care. Ultimately, providers' perspectives on what constitutes good practice could become transformed.

The larger system question is what should be provided as a part of health care. The current U.S. health care model equates health care with medical services. By that definition, a "Great Divide" defines what services are provided and where they are provided. Patients who are discharged from the hospital are no longer acutely ill by hospital criteria, but they are often still sick and weak from a functional and patient perspective. Even home health services are defined by skilled services, not by degree of dependency. While supportive services should rightfully be considered a part of health care, they are not a part of health services.

The demonstration sites showed that community care needs were clear and that the gap in services is evident. It was also evident from the strong response that the demonstration RFP received that many KP staff believed in this larger vision of health care. The demonstration projects showed that once a medical system and its providers understood and acknowledged that they were not attuned to community care needs and services, they could begin to consider the implications for their patients/members in terms of lack of information, frustration in seeking services, and ultimately, lower quality community care for frail members and high stress for caregivers.

Without raising consciousness of problems and solutions in these ways, it may not be possible to break down the institutional and professional barriers that have been built between medical and community care. And without breaking down those barriers, it may not be possible to turn around the over-medicalization of care. By giving medical care practitioners first-hand contact with the caregivers who make it possible to live day-to-day with disabilities, medical care may trust more to community care. And by addressing the weaknesses of community care, it will find more to trust. On both counts, people with disabilities and their family caregivers will be better served.

REFERENCES

Andersen, R., & Pourat, N. (1997). Toward a synthesis of a public health agenda for an aging society. In T. Hickey, M. Speers, & T. Prohaska (Eds.), *Public health and aging.* Baltimore: The Johns Hopkins University Press.

Capitman, J., & Sciegaj, M. (1995). A contextual approach for understanding individual autonomy in managed community long-term care. *Gerontologist, 35*(4), 533–540.

Greenlick, M. (1992). Educating physicians for population-based clinical practice. *Journal of the American Medical Association, 267*(12), 1645–1649.

8

A Prototype for 2005

Walter Leutz, Merwyn Greenlick, Richard DellaPenna, and Ed Thomas

---

The last chapter started with a review of the dire trends in disability demographics, medical care specialization, and community care marginalization, and it ended with high hopes for change through a community-oriented public health strategy led at least in part by linkage and coordination of the two systems. In between, the lessons from Manifesto 2005 demonstration sites showed that change will need to overcome numerous weaknesses in both systems, but the lessons also revealed strengths that seem capable of moving the systems in the right direction. Not the least of the strengths are people with disabilities themselves, who along with their families, generally find ways to put together the help they need—at times, in spite of the hassles thrown at them by the formal system.

Even if a community public health nirvana is unachievable, the situation could clearly be much better. This final chapter returns to the "here and now" and proposes practical prototypes for linkage and coordination of medical care and community care systems. The various demonstration projects that served distinct needs with particular services are merged into a more unified "mature" system that serves a range of member needs, and that connects with the complete constellation of community care services for each population of people with disabilities.

The demonstration experience gives every reason to think that these models are feasible, reasonable, and affordable. Although the mature models pose some challenges that were not encountered directly in the demonstration, the sites' experiences are still relevant. To discuss features of the models, some of the successful design features synthesized in chapters 2–6 are reviewed.

Mental model building is fun, but it does not address the question of where to get the financial support to test the models. Five years ago KP was ready to commit $3 million, but there is no assurance that this unusual source would be available today. What other sources could be tapped? Would expanding the demonstration to other organized medical systems and even fee-for-service settings also expand outside funding opportunities? From other health systems? Foundations? The federal government? From local communities themselves?

These questions inevitably lead back not just to practicality but to policy and politics. Assuming feasibility and affordability of the linkage and coordination model, is this the direction that key publics want to go? Are medical and community care organizations ready to cede some of their turf and resources to push for doing new jobs together? Are professionals willing to advocate for adding new dimensions and responsibilities to their jobs, while giving up some of their autonomy to others? Are policy makers and researchers who have pursued more sophisticated integration models of reform going to be convinced that simpler and less powerful approaches are worth trying? Can people with disabilities and their friends and families be enlisted to work with professionals and providers for a public health model when the ascendant ideology is to empower people by giving them cash to shop in the market? The book ends with some speculation on these points—but first a return to the practical.

PROTOTYPES FOR LINKAGE AND COORDINATION

Chapter 7 presented a series of lessons about linkage and coordination, from the points of view of the medical care system, the community care system, and service users. These won't be repeated here, but they are a useful reference in considering how to design and implement the details of the general models for linkage and coordination discussed in this chapter. This section reviews the structure, strengths, and weaknesses of the basic linkage model that was used by most demonstration sites and then outlines "mature" linkage and coordination models. After the quick overviews of the models, some of the features and their implications are elaborated.

The Typical Demonstration Model and its Shortcomings

Most service sites followed much the same linkage model (Figure 8.1). First, starting at the bottom of the figure, they worked with a particular community care service that members with disabilities could be using—e.g., community care "Program A" in the figure. Second, they set up a single point of contact (SPOC) in the medical care system to receive provider referrals and member inquiries, to handle communications with community agencies, and for general trouble shooting. Third, they trained medical care providers

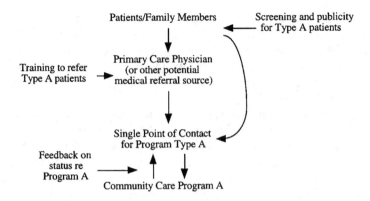

FIGURE 8.1 Typical demonstration model for linkage.

about the community service, how to refer to the SPOC, and which patients to refer. Fourth, they publicized the project to members through newsletters, flyers, and the like so that members could self-refer. Fifth, they established an information and tracking system to keep track of who was referred to the community care service and who got there. Not a great deal of new effort was required on the parts of linked community care agencies. They needed to give the time to educate health plan providers about their services and processes, to agree to consider referrals, and to let the health plan know if individuals were participating.

This design got most parts of the basic job done in the projects where it was tried. However, it was inefficient in at least three ways. First, with a few exceptions (the San Francisco, Vermont, and San Diego sites), projects had a relatively narrow focus on linking appropriate health plan members with a single community care service (e.g., adult day services, caregiver training). The single-service focus limited the relevance to members and providers but still required a full infrastructure of member outreach, provider training, and information systems.

Second, even when medical care providers tried to learn about community care services, they were often skeptical about their own ability to identify the people who might need a particular service. Now picture an expanded model that has separate linkage groups coming to providers and members "selling" their single services. Asking providers to distinguish who might be right for which one would almost certainly lead to the "your integration is my fragmentation" problem.

Several projects went beyond the single-service approach, and at least one seems to have had an easier "sell." The dementia project's agreement with the Alzheimer's Association was that the AA would pick up on all types of community care help that referred patients and caregivers might need. Providers seemed to be able to understand that there was something there for everyone, and they responded with referrals. The KP leadership in the San Diego service area combined three projects (dementia, community health workers, and volunteers) to create a multi-service approach to members with dementia and their caregivers. To manage this, they created a steering committee of clinical and management staff from all three projects. Finally, the San Francisco referrals project developed referral relationships with three types of agencies (personal care attendant, adult day services, and transportation) in order to have options to present to members who were referred. Thus, all three of these projects were able to tell referral sources, "we have a package," and to send people over for a discussion of what particular set of services might fit them best.

A third weakness in all service projects was limited, if any, member involvement in the design and evaluation of projects. Several projects (dementia, caregiver training, Vermont) used focus groups to identify member needs and program strengths and weaknesses, and these yielded valuable information. So did the satisfaction surveys conducted by these and some other projects. However, none went the next step of including service users actively in program design and ongoing review.

The Mature Linkage Model

The learning from the projects is synthesized in the "mature" linkage model pictured in Figure 8.2. Several features are added to the typical demonstration model. First, the core concept behind the mature model is that the SPOC expands its scope to include a broad range of community care programs for many if not all types of disability. This gives the SPOC the capacity to offer multiple options and to help people decide which is best for them.

Second, screening of and outreach to members are designed to reach all persons who have disabilities and who may want help better connecting with services. Outreach includes both general descriptions of the types of community care available, as well as highlights of particular types.

Third, training of physicians and other providers and care managers is more generic. Rather than giving providers multiple messages on numerous community care programs, training and information materials should be consolidated. The basic message is simpler and more powerful: engage patients and caregivers with apparent needs in a brief conversation followed by a strong message to contact the SPOC.[1]

---

[1] Of course, providers' primary responsibilities to these members are to provide their medical care and in the coordination model discussed presently, their responsibilities to coordinate medical care with community care are increased.

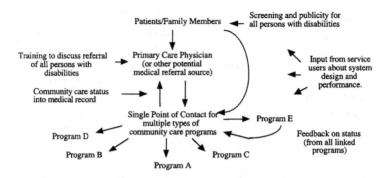

FIGURE 8.2   Mature linkage model.

The fourth addition to the mature linkage model that was on many agendas but not implemented in demonstration linkage sites is having information on functional status and caregiver issues (gathered by the SPOC and screening), and on community care status (from community agencies) in the medical record. This allows providers in any location to be alerted to functional status issues, to follow up on referrals to community care, to update participation in community care, and to inquire about informal caregivers.

The fifth addition is the inclusion of service users in the processes of designing and evaluating the system. This should include focus groups and satisfaction surveys, but it should go further. Both medical care and community care organizations can review current mechanisms and groups they have for user input and perhaps draw on existing systems. Enhancements will be needed, as discussed below.

The Coordination Model

Linkage may be as far as some medical care systems and community care systems can go, and it will serve many if not most persons with disabilities and their family caregivers well. But the demonstration showed that more was needed for people with more complex chronic illnesses, extensive community care needs, weak informal support or both. The most dramatic example was adult foster care home residents. They had inadequate support to bring them regularly to primary and preventive care visits; they required longer and more supported office visits than the health plan had available; their foster care providers did not have care links with the medical system beyond the prescription pad (and health plan providers were not able to give them more); and they had high rates of inpatient use that often bypassed the medical office. Another example was adult day services participants. There were service supports in day centers that demonstration sites wanted to use to support medical care plans.

To address these more intensive and individualized needs for cooperation between medical care and community care, we propose a "mature" coordination model. Although the day care and foster care sites had difficulty implementing all their plans, the plans that they made had most of the elements of coordination. Figure 8.3 adds these elements to the mature linkage model to illustrate a system with both linkage and coordination. First, the box shows that the relationship between medical care and a coordinated community care agency is formalized through a protocol that defines divisions of labor (particularly regarding case management and clinical plans of care), what services will be provided on what basis (e.g., eligibility, costs, procedures), and how communications about service status and clinical issues will be managed. This allows both community care and medical care to do more for individuals receiving coordination. Community care can receive up-to-date information about medical care issues and then support care at home—e.g., by helping with medication management, special diets, ambulation; by monitoring symptoms and changes; by making sure that medical appointments are kept and that there is transportation and escort if needed; and by phoning the SPOC with information and questions. Medical care enhances its own capabilities to include sharing up-to-date clinical information on nutrition, prescription drugs, and the like to community care; proactive tracking of admissions and discharges; special supports for ambulatory care visits (including longer visits); and sending medical providers to community care settings (e.g., foster care residents would be visited by health plan providers, as happens now with nursing home residents). Finally, medical care and community care may work together to identify and fill service gaps.

The left side of Figure 8.3 shows that these capabilities add another dimension to provider training and to the types of feedback providers receive about community care. Providers see not only that a patient is receiving community care, they see that a formal caregiver (rather than or in addition to an informal helper) is in the loop for medical care information and support.

Practical Lessons and Issues About Linkage and Coordination

Although none of the KP regions or service areas had enough projects to comprise a mature system of linkage and coordination, their experience is still relevant to design and implementation. Also, a few sites had more than one project, and, one service area combined projects to offer consolidated options to users.

The SPOC

The expanded responsibilities of the mature SPOC require some modification of approaches used in the demonstration. First, although the SPOC

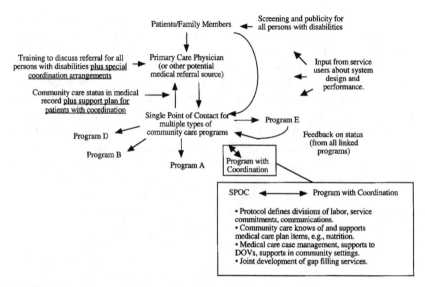

FIGURE 8.3   Mature linkage and coordination model.

looks generic from the outside, it likely makes sense for staff members with-in the SPOC to specialize in the needs and services for particular popula-tions, and it may even be wise to establish a separate point for certain groups—e.g., children with special needs, who would be seen mostly by pediatricians rather than adult-care physicians. Yet this cannot go too far; full specialization would create barriers, since a staff specialist may not be avail-able when a need arises.

Second, the physical and administrative location of the SPOC is an issue. The demonstration sites varied among continuing care (home health), social work, and geriatrics, in part reflecting who proposed the project. Any of these units might be appropriate in a particular organized medical care sys-tem. Another option that was not tried is member services. In any case, the unit needs to be near enough to clinical services to have close communica-tions with clinicians, but not so near as to be taken over by them, since actu-ally making community care connections is not part of medical providers' job. The unit also needs its own identity rather than having its tasks parcelled out. For example, the day care project found that the accomplishment of its activities was lost when they were diffused through the organization by hav-ing existing staffers devote a small portion of their time to them. And wher-ever the staff members are located, they will need good computer access and administrative support.

Third, the SPOC's interfaces with service users and professional staff need to be worked out. For example, the caregiver-training project had a recorded line for caregivers to call and ask either for written information about training or a callback to answer questions. They had a different line for providers to call to make referrals. In contrast, the dementia project had a single line staffed by a project professional for everyone to call. A generic SPOC will need to work out a triage system to handle a broader variety of calls from persons with disabilities and caregivers. Many of the calls will be easily dealt with by providing information, with the service user doing the follow-up, while other calls will require more direct assistance. Contacts from medical care providers and community agencies will likely need more consistent personal professional responses.

Relationships with Community Care Agencies

The SPOC staff will need linkage arrangements with the full range of community care programs in the core constellation of services for each population. A reasonable place to start for each population would be the following coordinating organizations: babies and children (early intervention), working age persons with physical disabilities (independent living centers), persons with intellectual disabilities (associations for retarded citizens), and aged with physical and cognitive disabilities (state and area agencies on aging). After contacting coordinating organizations, trade groups and individual local agencies could follow. Special connections to services related to particular conditions might also be warranted (e.g., multiple sclerosis, Alzheimers, cerebral palsy), as would connections to related advocacy and self-help groups.

The mature linkage and coordination models have implications for community care agencies and for the community care system as a whole. First, both supervisory and direct service staffs (especially in the coordination model) are asked to do extra work and more sophisticated work. Someone will need to pay for the additional supervision, information infrastructure, and training that would be required on the community care side. Second, exactly how community care staff providing coordinated services would work with the medical care system was barely explored in the demonstration. One issue is whether they would communicate with a community care supervisor, with the SPOC, with the physician, or with all three. Third, medical care would likely look to standardize information sharing and communications procedures with community care rather than negotiating each arrangement *de novo*. Fourth, the logic for better coordination among community care agencies becomes stronger. This could happen either through market models (preferred provider networks) or regulatory models (enhancement of publicly supported care coordination agencies). In short, once the medical system comes to count more on community care, it will likely expect more.

Provider Training

Training medical care providers how to work in a mature system poses new challenges and opportunities. On the one hand, the message from the SPOC to providers is simpler and stronger: "We can help with a broad range of needs related to disability—send us anyone about whom you have a question and we'll help them figure out what to do." The message to service users are similar: "Call us with your questions and we'll help you figure them out." On the other hand, there are nuances that can be added to those messages, and there are also some new capabilities to train providers to deal with.

Training medical care providers about patient needs and community care services and capabilities could be tailored to particular clinical concerns. Good examples of this are the demonstration sites' training of neurologists about the capabilities of the Alzheimers' Association protocol and of pediatricians about the early intervention connection. The San Francisco referral project envisioned going into detail: training physicians that a stroke patient can be maintained in adult day health care after rehabilitation by the health plan; teaching a physical therapist in home health that she or he can contact the adult day health physical therapist about what treatments have been used already; training a social worker to help a member under 60 to get home meals from a new program; training a nurse case manager to get a member with dementia subsidized respite care. Every discipline wouldn't be interested in all this detail, but each would want some. Training would need to walk a line between being so general that providers feel uninformed and being so specific that they are overloaded with information.

Providers would also need training in how to use new information in the medical record for patients who have already been identified by the SPOC. It would cover how to use the information about patient conditions and capabilities, caregivers, linkage opportunities and barriers, and current services. It would also explain how to update and add to the record. In systems that move into coordination, providers will need training on what populations are included, on the capabilities of coordination, and on the additional responsibilities they take on.

Outreach to Service Users

For many people who may need help with community care, "beating the bushes" is a more apt metaphor than "coming out of the woodwork." Therefore, outreach should be designed to catch the attention of people in various ways on the assumption that many will hesitate to seek help. Chapter 6 proposed a multi-level communication strategy to identify and reach potential service users in the population and to connect directly and smoothly with those who were interested. It included mass communication like posters and mailing inserts, information from members through surveys and focus groups, tailored communication such as program brochures, personalized communication such as provider discussions follow-up, service entry connections such as help lines and no-wait admission, and connections through service content and processes.

The mature linkage and coordination model maintains these approaches to reaching potential service users, but the content of the general messages changes. Overall, the public can be told that multiple product lines are available with one call, but, concurrently, each separate product line can continue to be "sold."

The expanded population focus in the mature model highlights the question of population screening. Medicare HMOs are required to screen all new members for risk factors, and most KP regions did this even before the 1997 requirements were passed. But there are no requirements for Medicare HMOs to re-screen members, for any screening of Medicare beneficiaries outside of managed care, or for screening of younger populations, where disability is less prevalent. Full population screening would be expensive (KP currently screens elders by mail at a cost of about $7 per person per year), so cheaper approaches to getting reliable and valid information are needed. At the request of KP's Care Management Institute, KP Aging Network, and all the divisions to bring the cost down for screening for common care-in-place syndromes and for identifying frail members, the Center for Health Research developed a Brief Health Questionnaire (BHQ) that costs $5 to send and process. The BHQ is ready for service in 2002. Another application of "real-time" screening is the new product called the Frailty Wheel. This is an interview tool using three questions and the member's age to quickly identify members at risk of being dependent on others for daily care. The demonstration's attempt to sift through administrative and clinical records showed the potential promise of an even cheaper system, but it was just a start.

Participation of Service Users

Participation of disabled people in system design must be real rather than window-dressing. This means not only providing seats on planning and oversight committees, but also developing infrastructures and procedures to make participation work. Inclusion regarding meeting times, transportation, accessibility, and communications are important. Both service users and professionals may need help. Supportive forums where service users and caregivers can meet to talk among themselves can be used to formulate positions that can be taken to larger bodies. Professionals may need process work to help them support changes in power relationships and procedures and to accept the authority deriving from the experience of service users. Ideally, the health plan, community care providers, and service users would work together to define issues, conduct research, and disseminate results in a participatory research model (Israel et al., 1998).

Information Systems

The mature linkage and coordination models have significant implications for information systems in both medical and community care. Most large medical systems have the technology to create some kind of "pop-up" item on the medical record to alert providers of community care issues and connections. The menu could prompt questions and allow addition of comments and updates. With provider training, the idea is, in a sense, to recreate "old Doc Smith," the mythical country doctor who knew everything about his patients, including their desired level of medical intervention through the end of life. For patients getting linkage, "Doc Smith" would know something about the family and community services. For patients getting coordination, his contacts would help him know what caregivers are doing and seeing.

Getting this information into the record requires routine input of (a) demographic and risk information from screening systems, (b) triggers for action based on high-risk status (as through KP's BHQ or Frailty Wheel screens), (c) referral information from the SPOC and other referrers, (d) service status information from community care providers (presumably fed through the SPOC), (e) comments from any provider involved with the service user, and (f) documents showing desired level of medical care intervention.

Achieving coordination requires three more types of information:

1. additional assessment information from case managers
2. care plan monitoring and support activities of community care providers, and
3. care plan information from medical care.

This is where the "rubber meets the road": Care plans should include specific things for the community care extension staff to check on and what to report back promptly if it changes. The medical record is closely guarded territory in medical care systems, and appropriately so. Making these kinds of changes will take both a consensus about their clinical importance and about the commitment of resources. It's easy to see why the demonstration sites made little progress on their small budgets and short timeframes.

The information system challenges to community care agencies are on a smaller scale, but even small changes and additions are daunting, given the lesser sophistication and smaller budgets in community care. Basic linkage requirements—informing medical care that a patient is participating—are a simple matter once release forms are in place and assuming the medical

SPOC is easy to reach. Coordination responsibilities are of a different order. They require obtaining and maintaining up-to-date clinical and care plan information from medical care, interpreting and transferring information and instructions to direct care workers (and it is likely to be more than one worker), receiving reports from workers, and transferring information back to medical care—all on a timely basis. At this point in the evolution of community care, some types of agencies (e.g., medical day care, foster care) will be more capable of doing this than others (e.g., home attendant care). Perhaps individuals needing coordinated home care can be served by more sophisticated agencies (e.g., home health), special arms of paraprofessional agencies, or extensions of medical care systems (as in the temporary decline and community health worker projects). The important point is that medical care should have information exchanges with whoever is in the supportive role for dependent members. This gets back to the broader definition of community care, including family, volunteers, neighbors, or the parish nurse.

Leadership and Location of Projects

The leadership and internal location of projects appeared to be important to their success. Things that helped included having a project leader with the power to keep it going, having a project that was congruent with existing roles and goals, being low-cost and integrated into existing operations and roles, having a physician champion, keeping visible, and forming a planning and oversight committee with the people who could help substantively and politically. Although service users weren't included in leadership, when they were tapped for focus groups and surveys, their input added not only substance but legitimacy.

Multi-site projects (e.g., dementia care, caregiver training, adult day services, and volunteers) had a number of advantages. They fostered team building, stronger protocol development, higher profiles for projects, and evaluation plans. There were challenges to coordination and extra costs from meeting, but there were offsetting savings from sharing core administrative support, consultants, and production of materials. Multi-site projects also had built-in replication tests. If an approach can work at multiple sites in a system, it disarms skeptics who say that it worked in the demonstration site(s) because they were special. Even in a single corporate system like KP, there are many differences in structure and process that could either enhance or inhibit adoption.

Summary

The demonstration sites showed that it is possible to link medical care and community care systems, and they did it over and over again on small

budgets and in short time frames. They didn't always get all the pieces working, but sometimes they did. There weren't always large flows of service
users, but sometimes there were. Medical care clinicians didn't always participate as hoped, but sometimes they did. The same could be said for community care providers. So linkage is feasible for the medical care system that
decides to do it, and community care agencies are ready to cooperate.

It is clear on many counts that linkage poses far fewer challenges for both
medical care and community care than does coordination. The former is a
relatively big step for medical care and a small one for community care.
Medical care needs to get its act together to recognize disability, talk to agencies in the community that can help, talk to patients about it, and try to help
them get connected to help. Community care just needs to be there in the
forms it's in now.

Coordination was another matter. The sites did not prove the feasibility
of coordination, but they did identify pressing needs for this kind of help—
among foster care residents, post-acute patients, and persons with dementia.
More individuals could have been identified in all projects. Although they
fell short of implementing the coordination model, the approaches that sites
tried to implement made sense, as synthesized and presented above. The
question is not so much whether it is feasible to coordinate medical and community care as we have described, but rather on what terms, particularly
what cost.

NEXT STEPS

Most of the demonstration projects ended or greatly scaled back their linkage and coordination activities with the end of funding. Without explicit
support, it was difficult to staff the single point of contact, maintain up-to-
date community contacts, and train providers without explicit support.
Some activities continued, however, particularly at the multi-site projects.
The dementia sites continued to follow the post-diagnosis protocol, as did
the participating Alzheimers Associations. Most of the caregiver training and
volunteer sites continued, albeit it on a scaled-back basis given reduced outreach. The foster care project and one of the day care sites moved into a second phase. That's not a bad record, but KP certainly has the makings to do
more. The ideas and most of the people that made the demonstration happen
are still there and ready for more. Many people like them exist across the
medical care and community care systems.

Kaiser Permanente is taking stock of the experience and considering its
own next steps. This manuscript and an executive summary were sent to
KP's administrative and medical leadership, its relevant inter-regional planning bodies (e.g., the Care Management Institute, the KP Aging Network),

the Garfield Memorial Fund, as well as the leaders of each of the demonstration projects. As of this writing, they are considering options and setting priorities through existing procedures.

There are many compelling reasons for KP to continue to work on linkage and coordination. The linkage and coordination models tested in the demonstration are consistent with established KP elder care and disability care programs. For example, the Eldercare Source Book produced by the Care Management Institute reviews the importance of medication management, transition support, end of life care, nursing facility care, and screening for members with chronic illnesses and functional limitations. But it does not include any processes or infrastructure to connect to the community care supports that are essential to make them work for many patients. A linkage and coordination system would have similar synergy with the model of care's medical case management, the SEEK system's identification of functional impairments and need for help with community care, the Cooperative Health Care Clinics' support groups for high-use members, and the KP Promise to "know us as members, and provide us with personalized, top quality medicine, with great service."

The KP system may decide to pursue an expanded test on its own, but KP also supported a public domain evaluation of the demonstration because leaders believe the demonstration has broader relevance. It is hoped that other organized medical systems and communities will consider following suit and that national funders will also be interested. A multi-HMO demonstration in several communities would be a great way to learn more.

The linkage and coordination model could also be tested in a community operating in a fee-for-service environment. A rural area is an obvious choice, since both medical care and community care systems would be relatively simple. But workable models can also be conceived in more urban areas. A starting point might be to extend the British and U.S. "attached nurse" medical screening and case management models discussed in chapter 1 (Williams n.d.) to include linkage to community care care. A single point of contact could serve multiple medical practices and also be connected with hospitals' and nursing homes' discharge departments, as well as with skilled home health agencies.[2]

Success of either HMO or fee-for-service initiatives on the medical care side would depend in large part on the strength of the community care system in terms of both services and organization. Linkage to community care services would be easier in states systems or both with a single point of entry for community care services. Linkage would be more successful in states or

---

[2] Old hands in long-term care may recognize a resemblance to Ruchlin, Morris, and Eggert's Local Area Management Organization (LAMO). A key difference is that the LAMO was based not on referral relationships but on taking over financing and case management.

systems with adequate services (e.g., assisted transportation for foster care residents, respite for caregivers attending support and training classes). Other elements that would help would be adequate community care staffing, supervision, and cross-training resources. These are the kinds of things that could be enhanced through demonstration funds and local enhancements.

CONCLUDING THOUGHTS

This demonstration showed that linkages between HMOs and community care services are feasible and affordable. But these results are preliminary; without more rigorous tests, many observers will remain unconvinced of the model's capacity to improve outcomes, offset costs with savings, or even improve access for members. Only broader and deeper tests will provide clearer answers.

A great deal is being invested in new medical models for chronic illness care and new financing and delivery models for integrated acute and long-term care. Devising and testing these more profound changes in the delivery of care will take time and resources, and the results are uncertain. They rely on organized health systems being ready to take risk for new and complex business ventures in partnership with public agencies. In the meantime, the more modest linkage model could move quickly to fill service and coordination gaps for a broad range of persons with chronic illnesses and disabilities. Where full integration works, it can always be folded in on top of linkage and coordination.

In endorsing and testing Manifesto 2005, KP once again displayed its leadership in health policy. It led the way because of what it is and because it can. In organizing and implementing the demonstration, KP showed some of the characteristics that distinguish it from other health systems, and that distinguish medical care from community care. It mustered national funding and planning capabilities to start the demonstration, and it implemented through established local service area administrative and communications systems (e.g., forming planning teams, expanding jobs of the existing staff, training through grand rounds and departmental meetings, communicating through batch email and newsletters). Even with the systems and resources the health plan had to implement change, it was not easy to move large systems.

The KP system now needs to decide if this is a health plan priority. That is, should linkage and coordination be system benefits? Are they consistent with what the health plan wants to be for its members in the long term? Will they be included as part of the KP Promise? Will other health systems follow suit? If KP goes forward and competitors do not, will KP stand out as a winner that was ahead of the curve or a holdover from an idealistic public health past that cannot meet market tests?

Innovation in expanding services and coordination across systems would certainly be easier if there were a national policy framework for stronger and more widespread linkages. To foster compliance with the Supreme Court's decision on Olmstead vs. Georgia, Congress recently mandated and funded state initiatives in "Real Choices" to strengthen community care infrastructure. Will the state projects include linkage and coordination initiatives or continue to develop community care systems segregated from medical care? Is a new and separate initiative for linkage needed? Another approach would be for Medicare to add a linkage payment increment to HMOs and even PCPs with linkage (for under 65 disabled too). This would be consistent with a vision of Medicare that promotes maintaining function in addition to treating illness (Greenlick, 1996).

While national initiatives from the medical care side are needed, they won't get too far without a concomitant investment in community care services. The difficulties in access and gaps in service encountered at demonstration sites reflect the reality that there are many, many people with disabilities in the United States who are not getting all the help they need at home and in their communities. We need to invest more in public services to help them. This is an issue that cuts across the integration/coordination/linkage question. You can't integrate a service that does not exist, nor can you link with it.

This brings the question back to the politics of public and professional support for how and how much help is provided to persons with disabilities. It may be possible to change politics if the system is moving in the direction of changes in how to conceive, deliver, and guide services. The key may be to look to the community as the locus of the system. The concept is community-based public health that is less medicalized, delivered in home and community settings, coordinated across systems, and guided by user preferences in design and services delivered. The demonstration experience lends credence to the idea that community stakeholders—providers, government, professionals, and citizens—can come together to make change.

Many may be skeptical of the feasibility of community initiatives, particularly in a time when individualistic and market-oriented solutions are in the ascendancy. In comparing long-term care in the United States to that Canada, Clark, (1991) observed: "Strait jacketed by . . . individualism, [Americans] are unable to engage in any meaningful public dialogue on what the goals of society should be and the appropriate means for achieving them. . . . We substitute economic incentives and cost-cutting procedures for real social dialogue in the vain hope that these will solve what is at heart a crisis of shared values and principles. . . ." But there is another side to that character that also can be tapped. Given the activist histories of disability communities, the state and local control of disability policy, the profusion of voluntary agencies, and the widespread involvement of families in caregiving, a pro-community policy could nurture and structure that involvement and create a coalition that can transform the system and sustain it with effective political support. These are big visions, but vision is needed to address the clear challenges of aging and disability in society.

REFERENCES

Brody, K., Johnson, R. E., & Ried, D. L. (1997). Evaluation of a self-report screening instrument to predict frailty outcomes in aging populations. *The Gerontologist, 37*(2), 182–191.

Clark, P. G. (1991). Ethical dimensions of quality of life in aging: Collectivism in the United States and Canada. *The Gerontologist, 31*(5), 631–639.

Greenlick, M. (1996). The house that Medicare built: Remodeling for the 21st century. *Health Care Financing Review, 18*(2), 131–145.

Israel B. A., Schulz, A. J., Parker, E. A., & Becker, A. B. (1998). Review of community-based research: Assessing partnership approaches to improve public health. *Annual Review of Public Health, 19,* 173–202.

Williams, F. n.d. The John A. Hartford Generalist Physician Initative Report. Tempe, AZ: Arizona State University School of Health Administration and Policy.

Index

Springer Publishing Company

Effective Health Behavior in Older Adults

K. Warner Schaie, PhD,
Howard Leventhal, PhD,
Sherry L. Willis, PhD, Editors

In what ways do health behaviors and societal mechanisms help or discourage individuals in assuming responsibility for their health? Highly-esteemed and diverse contributors examine the health behaviors of older adults and the ways in which these behaviors are affected by societal trends.

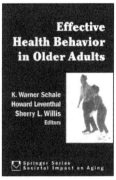

The volume begins with a discussion of the personal attributes affecting health behaviors and responsible health care choices in older adults. Additional topics explored include: psychosocial factors in the prevention of cardiovascular disease; behavioral interventions such as the role of exercise in preventing chronic illness; and how societal structures such as reimbursement patterns and changes in health insurance affect initiation, change, and maintenance of health behaviors.

Partial Contents:

- Biosocial Considerations in Chronic Illness Perceptions and Decisions, *T. Hickey*
- Linear and Dynamical Thinking about Psychosocial Factors and Cardiovascular Risk, *J. Suls and R. Martin*
- Commentary: Acute and Chronic Psychological Processes in Cardiovascular Disease, *D.W. Johnston*
- Psychosocial Factors in the Prevention of Cardiovascular Disease, *L.H. Powell*
- Ethnicity and Psychosocial Factors in Cardiovascular Disease Prevention, *K.E. Whitfield, T.A. Baker, and D.T. Brandon*
- Getting Help to Those Most Likely to Benefit: Patient Characteristics and Treatment Success, *J.C. Barefoot*
- Exercise Interventions and Aging, *J.A. Blumenthal and E.C.D. Gullete*
- Commentary: Challenges to using Exercise Interventions in Older Adults, *E.A. Burns*

Springer Series on Societal Impact on Aging
2002   344pp   0-8261-2401-1   hard $49.95 (outside US $54.80)

536 Broadway, New York, NY 10012 • 212-431-4370 • Fax: 212-941-7842
Order Toll-Free: 877-687-7476 • www.springerpub.com

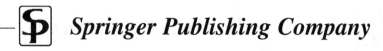

Springer Publishing Company

Dementia and Wandering Behavior
Concern for The Lost Elder
Nina M. Silverstein, PhD, Gerald Flaherty,
Terri Salmons Tobin, PhD

Professionals and family caregivers need to know that there are preventive measures available to create safer environments that maximize autonomy while minimizing risk for people with dementia in their care.

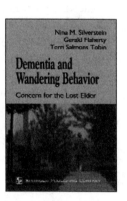

Authors Silverstein, Flaherty, and Tobin focus on specific responses to wandering behavior, and describe ways to create a safe environment in the home, community, and care facility. Written in a clear and accessible style, this book draws attention to a life-threatening problem facing an estimated two to four million Americans.

Partial Contents:

Part I: Introduction
- Alzheimer's Disease and Related Dementias: An Overview
- Comprehensive Review of the Literature on Wandering Behavior

Part II: Current Community Responses to Wandering Behavior, What Works, What Doesn't, and Why?
- Law Enforcement, Technology
- Community Service and Long Term Care Providers

Part III: Creating a Safe Environment
- The Home: Recommendations for Family Caregivers
- The Facility: Recommendations for Long Term Care and Assisted Living Residences
- The Community: Recommendations for Elder Care and Acute Care Providers
- The Lifesaving Role of "First Responders": Recommendations for Police, EMS, Fire, and Search & Rescue Personnel

2002   232pp   0-8261-4262-1   soft $37.95 (outside US $42.80)

536 Broadway, New York, NY 10012 • 212-431-4370 • Fax: 212-941-7842
Order Toll-Free: 877-687-7476 •   www.springerpub.com